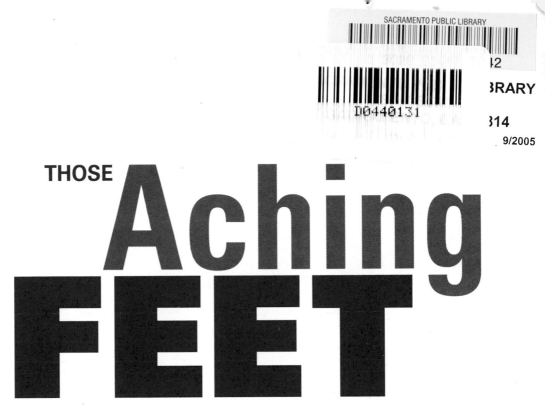

THOSE Aching FEET

Your Guide to Diagnosis and Treatment of Common Foot Problems

Revised Edition

Dr. Christine Dobrowolski
Doctor of Podiatric Medicine

SKI
PUBLISHING

Those Aching Feet:
Your Guide to Diagnosis and Treatment of Common Foot Problems
Revised Edition

Special acknowledgement to my dad and his numerous foot problems

Special thanks to: Jay, Joe, Pam, Mom, and Lawrence

First published by SKI Publishing, 2004
This revised edition published by SKI Publishing, 2005

Published by SKI Publishing Co.
302 Balboa Street, San Francisco, CA 94118
mail@SKIpublishing.com
www.SKIpublishing.com

ISBN 0-9654612-2-X
Library of Congress Control Number: 2003095214

Published in the United States of America
Printed in the United States of America

DISCLAIMER: It is not the intention of this book to substitute for a visit to your health care provider. We will not be held liable for any diagnosis made or treatment rendered. Consult your doctor if you feel you have a medical problem.

None of the registered, trademarked or copyrighted names included in this book were meant to slander or in any way demean the name, product or company associated with, and cannot be misinterpreted or misrepresented to alter this. Including, but not limited to: Advil®, Aldara®, alpha-lipoic acid (ALA), American Orthopedic Foot and Ankle Society, baclofen®, Bextra®, Burrows®, Canthacur®, capsacian, Celebrex®, cimetidine, Daypro®, Desenex®, Elavil®, epsom salt, Extracorporeal Shock Wave Therapy, Feldene®, Fletch, free-radicals, Gamma linolenic acid (GLA), Kerasal®, ketamine, ketoprofen, KOH, Lamisil®, Lotrimin®, Mobic®, Morton's neuroma, Motrin®, Naprosyn®, National Shoe Retailers Association, Neurontin®, Pedorthic Footwear Association, pedorthists, Penlac®, podiatrist, Prexige®, Reiter's syndrome, Relafen®, Sporonox®, Tagamet®, tea tree oil, terfenadine, Tinactin®, Tylenol®, Vioxx®, Zostrix®.

I am dedicating this book to my grandad who passed away due to complications from diabetes.

Contents

INTRODUCTION

Chapter Overview

I wanted to write a book about common foot problems because I have found that many people ignore their feet. I see patients with foot problems who will wait six months to a year before seeking treatment. Many times, early treatment can help avoid further complications or eventual surgery. This book is designed to help you recognize foot disorders, learn how to start treatment yourself and to help you understand when it is necessary to see a physician.

The first chapter concentrates on foot definitions and anatomy. It's your orientation about the foot. The basic design of the remaining chapters of the book is simple. Each chapter is titled with the common layman terminology. For instance, Chapter 1 is "Fungal Nails". Underneath the title is the medical terminology "onychomycosis". The **Overview** at the beginning of the chapter will introduce the reader to the condition and give some background on the condition. How often the condition occurs and why it occurs will be explained.

The second section is **What You See and Feel**. It describes what you may see on your foot and what types of sensations you feel, for instance pain, itching or cramping. The medical terminology for this description would be "signs and symptoms."

The next section in each chapter will discuss **How It's Diagnosed**. A diagnosis gives a name to the disease, process or condition that is affecting you. This section will discuss how the diagnosis is made and what type of tests may or may not be needed.

What Else Could It Be? is a question most people ask after they are given their diagnosis. There are usually, but not always, other conditions to be considered. What this means to you is for a specific complaint, there may be more than one possible diagnosis to consider. For example, a painful thick yellow nail is most likely a "fungal nail", but the doctor may need to consider other conditions like psoriasis or a bruising injury. Other conditions common in the area with similar symptoms need to be considered when making the final diagnosis. Tests may need to be ordered to make the final diagnosis, or it may be as simple as a quick exam or good questioning. It all depends on the condition.

The next section in each chapter will tell you **What You Can Do About It**. This will discuss the best treatment options for you. I do not discuss all of the treatments for each condition, rather I focus on the most effective and most common treatments. In this section I may suggest a visit to your physician, and sometimes I will provide you with questions to ask your physician. If you have any questions regarding the treatments presented, or if you are unsure if the medications mentioned should be taken with your current medications, consult your physician.

Some sections will list the **Side Effects** of the medications that I have discussed or complications with the procedures I mention. At the end of each chapter, I will present **The Bottom Line**; a short summary of the chapter's important points. This area is a good reference if you want to look up information quickly.

Some words are *italicized* to let you know that a complete definition of that word is located in the glossary at the back of the book.

1

Anatomy and Terms

Overview

Medical terminology can be very confusing. It's riddled with obscure, funny looking words that are often long and difficult to pronounce. Some terms may be familiar, while others are not. Other times you will see a word that is familiar to you, but you are not exactly sure what it means. This chapter will give a basic overview of the anatomy of the foot and some basic terms used to describe the foot's function. In this chapter and throughout the book, drawings are provided to assist you in understanding the terminology.

Anatomy

There are 28 bones in the foot and over a hundred ligaments. The foot also has tendons, muscles, blood vessels and nerves.

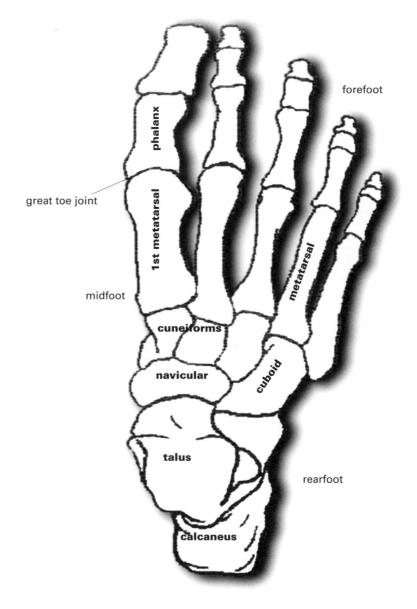

forefoot

phalanx

great toe joint

1st metatarsal

metatarsal

midfoot

cuneiforms

navicular

cuboid

talus

rearfoot

calcaneus

Figure 1-1 bones of the foot

The heel bone is also called the calcaneus. The bone
that sits on top of the heel bone and is part of the ankle
joint is called the talus. The bone that sits in front of the
heel bone is called the cuboid. These bones make up
the rearfoot. The bones in the middle of the foot (also

Those Aching Feet

called the midfoot) are called cuneiforms and the navicular. The long bones in the foot, that extend to the front of the foot are metatarsals. These metatarsals are numbered from one to five, starting with the largest on the inside of the foot in the arch area. The bones in the toes are phalanges. There are 14 phalanges in each foot. The last two bones are small bones that sit under the first metatarsal. These bones are called sesamoids, they act as lever arms and assist with tendon function. These bones make up the forefoot. The "great toe joint" is the

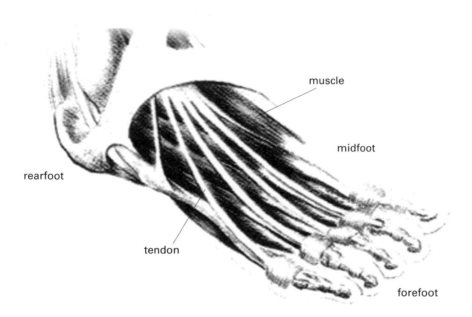

Figure 1-2 anatomy of the foot

common term for the meeting of the first metatarsal and the largest phalanx.

A *ligament* is a band like structure that is made up mostly of collagen and attaches from one bone to another, usually crossing a joint. A *tendon* is a fibrous

1: Anatomy and Terms   7

band in tubular form that attaches muscle to bone. Blood vessels can be arteries or veins. *Arteries* bring blood with oxygen and nutrients from the heart to the rest of the body. *Veins* bring the blood from the rest of the body back to the heart. *Capillaries* are at the junction between the arteries and the veins. This is the point where the oxygen and the nutrients can transfer from the blood vessels to the tissues. Fibrous tissue is a connective tissue (connects one structure to another). This tissue is similar to scar tissue, and is made of collagen.

Terminology

Medial means placed towards the center of the body. *Lateral* means away from the middle of the body. *Pronation* is a motion of the foot that is difficult to describe. Start by thinking of the ankle sitting directly on top of the heel. In pronation, the ankle shifts towards the center of the body as the heel turns away

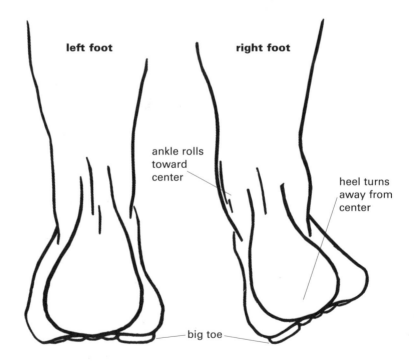

Figure 1-3 pronation (eversion)

Those Aching Feet

from the body (see Figure 1-3). *Supination* is the opposite of pronation; the ankle is shifting away from the center of the body and the heel turns toward the center. These are difficult terms to understand. To better understand this motion, use yourself as an example. Stand up, keep both feet in place and rotate your body around to the left, looking over your left shoulder. The left foot will be supinated and the right foot will be pronated. I will also mention two other terms that are actually separate and different movements, but for the purposes of the this book consider them the same as the above mentioned motions. *Eversion* is comparable to pronation. *Inversion* is comparable to supination.

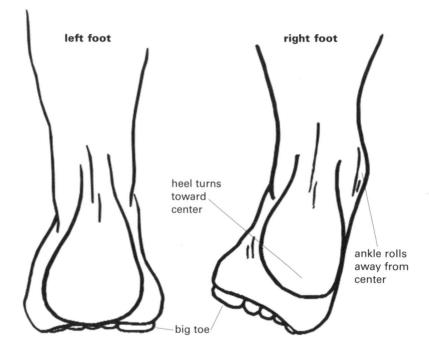

left foot

right foot

heel turns
toward
center

ankle rolls
away from
center

big toe

Figure 1-4 supination (inversion)

2

Fungal Nails
on·y·cho·my·co·sis

Overview

Fungal nails are a problem that affect between 5 to 25% of the population. All ages can be affected, but it's most commonly seen developing in those between the ages of 40-60 years and the percentage increases with age. In the 1800s, fungal nails were very rare. The increased prevalence is linked to the increase in exposure to fungus through the use of showering facilities in gyms, spas, saunas and pools. More individuals are playing sports, wearing occlusive footwear and the general population has aged. The increase is also linked to those who are *immunocompromised*. This includes those with diabetes and HIV and those taking medications that suppress the immune system for diseases like rheumatoid arthritis and cancer. Some individuals have a higher chance of getting fungal nails. These include

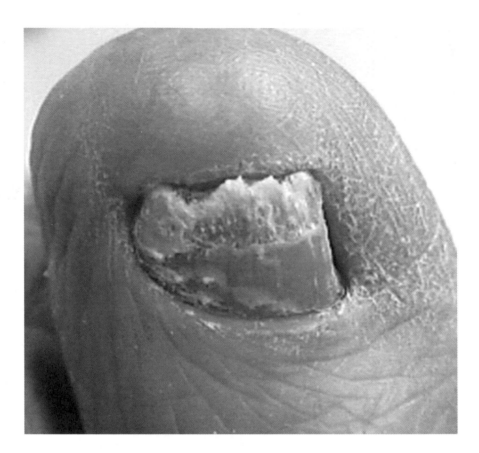

Figure 2-1 Thick yellow nail with brittle edges represents a classic fungal nail of the great toe.

elderly people, people with diabetes and people whose immune systems don't function normally. When the immune system is not working at full force, the fungus has an easier time invading. As we get older, the collagen bonds that form the skin layers become weaker. It is a slow process, but when they become weak and have microscopic openings, it gives the fungus an opportunity to invade and cause an infection. Some individuals inherit the unique susceptibility to fungal infections and may get the fungus at a young age regardless of their health. No matter who you are, no matter how healthy you are, once the fungus has gotten into your nails, it is extremely difficult to remove.

What You See and Feel

The first evidence of the fungus usually is white lines (longitudinal lines) in the nail, sometimes with white splotchy areas. The nail becomes an unusual shape and can appear lumpy or irregular. Other signs include yellow patches or thickening, and sometimes there can be a dark brown discoloration. As the disease progresses, the nails become thicker and tend to grow up instead of growing out. The fungus actually invades the *nail bed* (skin layer below the nail that tells the nail how to grow) and this affects the shape of the nail. Fungal nails can be brittle, hard, flakey, firm or ingrown (Figure 2-1).

How It's Diagnosed

To determine if the nail has a fungus, your physician may do a test called a *KOH*. This preparation allows physicians to look under the microscope for *hyphae* (spaghetti like structures indicating the microscopic appearance of a fungus). This is not always needed, because most fungal nails can be diagnosed by a physician simply by evaluating the nail. In fact, most patients know what they have before they walk into the doctor's office. But, in the case of uncertainty, you may find some physicians doing this test. Some insurance companies may require a KOH before authorizing treatment.

What Else Could It Be?

There are a number of other things that could be affecting the nails, but I will only name a few because 99% of the time it is a fungus. When the nails take on a darker appearance, or have a white patchy look, there may be another underlying disease.

A physician might consider malignant melanoma, psoriasis or nail bruising. Malignant melanoma is rare and almost never looks like a fungus, but in the case of a darkened area under the nail without a history of injury, further evaluation may be justified. The area below the nail can be evaluated and possibly biopsied.

Another possible diagnosis is psoriasis. The pitting in the nails and white lines can commonly look like fungus and actually be psoriasis. Long term exposure to water can also cause the nails to look like they are affected by a fungus. Repetitive microtrauma, common in runners, can also result in thickened and discolored nails that appear like a fungus. Remember that most of the time it's fungus.

What You Can Do About It

There are many treatments for fungal nails ranging from over-the-counter remedies to prescriptions for oral medications.

Starting with the most conservative treatment, a home remedy that works is using bleach.
- A small amount of bleach can be applied to the nail with a toothbrush or q-tip after roughening the surface with a nail file. Let it sit for five minutes then rinse.
- Use this twice a day, every day, for approximately six months.
- With diligent application, the yellowish thickening may decrease, but the fungus will most likely not resolve completely.
- Stop using if you notice skin irritation from the bleach.
- Do not soak your feet in bleach.

Another home-treatment is tea tree oil.
- Tea tree oil has been shown to be effective against fungus.
- Tea tree oil can be effective if used properly.
- About six months of twice a day applications need to be done for full effectiveness.
- Chances of 100% resolution are slim with this treatment.

There are some preparations available at the drug store that maybe be effective.
- These treatments will be unlikely to remove the fun-

A 45 year old mother of two presented to me with a complaint of fungal nails. She described her nails, as she showed me, they were thickened, white and flakey at the ends. She described parts of the nail just peeling off. After trying different types of anti-fungal medications on her, and failing, I questioned her about her nail cleaning habits. She stated that she was "extremely good about cleaning her nails, filing them every day, lifting the edges to avoid ingrown nails, and soaking the feet twice a day." After further questioning, I found that she soaked her feet about 1 hour at a time, also took baths, and used the hot tub. In her meticulous process of nail care, she tended to peel the layers of nails off after soaking. She diligently applied the anti-fungal solutions three to four times a day in large amounts. Basically, she was overdoing everything and water-logging her nails. The nails would then separate and would peel and appear flakey and dry. After discontinuing her meticulous approach to her feet, she slowly improved. Without any medication her nails were back to normal in four weeks.

gus completely and it is my experience that they are about 5-20% effective.
- Be sure to buy an anti-fungal nail product in a solution or a spray.
- Some patients have reported results with Vicks Vapor Rub®, but I have found limited success with this.

Prescription topicals are the next option.
- Although the companies may boast high efficacy rates, I have found them to be about 20-30% effective.
- Part of this low efficacy rate is due to lack of patient compliance. This means that it is difficult to apply the medication daily for six to eight months.
- Another reason is that with any topical, it is difficult for the medication to penetrate through the nail to the nail bed.
- One prescription topical is Penlac®. Penlac® is the best of the prescription topical nail anti-fungal medications. It has been been shown to be quite effective in decreasing the yellow discoloration and thickness.

Oral anti-fungal medications are effective but have side effects.
- The two common oral anti-fungal medications are Sporonox® and Lamisil® (Lamisil® is both a topical

and an oral medication.)

- These two medications are much safer than the older anti-fungal medications, which had significant toxic effects on the liver.
- Both of these anti-fungal medications involve three months of daily or weekly therapy (depending on the medication).
- Baseline blood tests are done on the liver since these medications have been shown to have a 3-7% chance of increasing the liver enzymes. These effects are minimal, and the tests are usually done only once.
- If an individual is taking a blood thinner or has liver problems, the liver is monitored on a monthly basis.
- These medications are taken for three months, but they will stay in the nail while the nail grows out over the next 8-12 months.
- The medications range in effectiveness from 60-80%.
- There is still a chance of re-infection after finishing the course of the medication. The re-infection rate is 15%, but can be as high as 25% in diabetics.
- Serious adverse reactions are less than 0.5%.
- There are some interactions between these medications and other drugs that you may be taking; such as cyclosporine, cimetidine, rifampin, terfenadine, and caffeine.

I only recommend oral therapy to those people who are having pain or who are having chronic infections as a result of the fungal nails. I also recommend it to diabetics with loss of sensation who do not have any drug interactions. This is to help resolve the fungal infection before the nails becomes severely deformed and causes ingrown nails. Diabetics have a higher chance of reinfection even if the therapy is successful.

I recommend to many patients to take a "preventative care" approach. Many people are intimidated or 'turned off' by the twice daily routine of topical therapy. I recommend using a topical once a week or a few times a month to prevent the fungus from getting

Children

There have been no FDA studies on the oral anti-fungal medications in children. The studies that have been done, mostly involve fungal skin infection, not fungal nail infections. These studies required only one to four weeks of the medications, not the twelve weeks necessary for toenails. The studies done have had few patients, but the side effects and complications are minimal and rare.

Side Effects

The side effects are rash, abdominal pain, constipation, diarrhea, headache, taste disturbances. Those patients that had abnormal liver test results due to the medication, in general did not experience any problems. The lab tests returned to normal as soon as the medication was stopped. Serious adverse effects include hepatitis and acute hepatic necrosis

worse. This will not treat the nail, but may help prevent the spread and progression.

The Bottom Line

Are you having pain or infections as a result of the fungal nails? Are you diabetic and have a loss of sensation? Then you are a candidate to take the oral medications. If not then I would recommend starting with topical therapy. You need to consider the possible side effects and the cost of the medication. Both of these medications usually run about $600 to $700 for three months. If you are lucky, your insurance will pay for some of it. For the really severe cases, or individuals that have been very resistant to one of the drugs or the other, I recommend removing the nail (nail avulsion), taking oral therapy and using topicals.

3

Ingrown Nails
on·y·cho·cryp·to·sis

Overview

An ingrown nail is a nail that curves into the skin. It may be painful, and may cause infection. An ingrown nail that causes infection or inflammation is called a paronychia. Ingrown nails or *onychocryptosis*, can be caused by a variety of things. Trauma, or any damage to the nail or the nail bed can result in ingrown nails. This can be blunt trauma, like dropping something on your toe, or microtrauma, repetitive pressure on your toes. Military cadets in basic training will commonly have ingrown toenails. Runners, tennis players and especially kids starting new sports like soccer or football commonly have ingrown toenails. There is the infamous fungus that can cause ingrown nails. Any time the nail is removed it can regrow as an ingrown nail. Some people naturally have curved nails that have

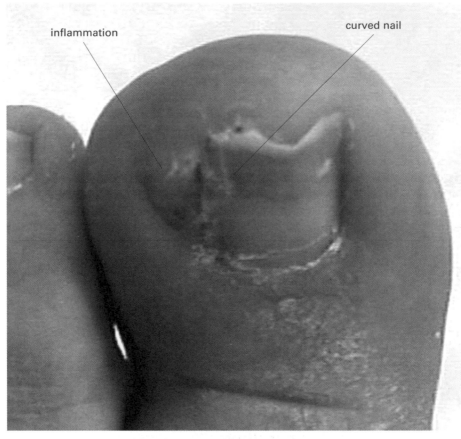

inflammation

curved nail

Figure 3-1 Ingrown Nail

a tendency to turn in. Rigid shoes, new shoes and narrow shoes can cause ingrown nails. A new activity can result in an ingrown nail. Cutting the nail along the border can sometimes result in ingrown nails. Lastly, a bone spur can cause an abnormal growth and result in an ingrown nail.

What You See and Feel

An ingrown nail has a curved look to it. It can be subtle or it can be severe. Most fungal ingrown nails are fairly severe. It may cause redness, swelling, drainage and a significant amount of pain. It may only cause pain, and may not be very swollen or red. In any of these cases, treatment will be required.

How To Diagnose It

There is no diagnostic test for an ingrown nail. Most people, physician or layman, can tell if a nail is ingrown. It is difficult though to tell whether the toe is infected or only inflamed. It is commonly inflamed when it is red and swollen, but not always infected.

What Else Could It Be?

There are very few other things it could be. If the nail is raised centrally and severely curved on the sides, then sometimes it is necessary to take an x-ray to make sure that a bone spur is not causing the nail deformity. This is not common, but with some nails it must be considered. There can be other things under the nail that may cause an ingrown nail which would require nail removal, but these are also rare.

What You Can Do About It

There are about five options for treatments for ingrown nails.

The first option is to trim the sides of the nails.
- Gives temporary relief without requiring an injection of *anesthesia* (numbing medication).
- Combined with soaking, this will help the athlete through a training session or a basketball or soccer game.
- This can provide relief for someone until a more permanent procedure can be done.

The second option is antibiotics.
- Many physicians will prescribe antibiotics to decrease the swelling and redness before the patient sees their podiatrist.
- This treatment may also only be temporary for many patients.

The third option is a *partial nail avulsion*.

- This procedure requires anesthesia and removes only the side of the nail that is causing a problem.
- The side of the nail is removed all of the way to the nail root.
- This will allow the swelling and redness to decrease.
- It will take 8-12 months for the nail to grow back in completely.
- The goal is to obtain a normal nail when it regrows.
- About fifty percent of the time it will regrow incorrectly, this varies considerably on the type of nail.
- The nail appears in one to two months. If it's ingrown there will be pain and redness following in two to four months.
- I recommend this treatment to those who don't have chronic problems with ingrown nails
- I also recommend it to those who developed the ingrown nail as a direct result of a pair of shoes or sports/athletic activity.

The next option is called a *partial matrixectomy*.
- This means that the side of the nail is taken, not the entire nail, and a chemical is used to kill the nail root (called the *matrix*).
- The chemical will not allow the nail to regrow. Therefore, part of the nail will be missing, and the end result is a more narrow nail.
- About 5-10% of the time, the nail will regrow.
- This treatment is best for those who have chronic ingrown nail problems and those who have deformities of the nail bed. When the nail bed is deformed (for instance, as a result of fungus or an injury) then the nail will always regrow incorrectly.
- Those individuals with very poor circulation, as diagnosed by a physician, should not have this procedure done.
- This is a great procedure for diabetics with good blood flow. It will help to avoid future problems.
- If an individual has poor blood supply or has been resistant to the chemicals used, then the matrix can be removed surgically. This involves cutting it out and sewing up the toe.

Post Surgery Care

It is not recommended to put on topical antibiotics after these procedures, it will block drainage. The drainage needs to come out in order to decrease inflammation. Do not do this unless your physician instructs you to do so.

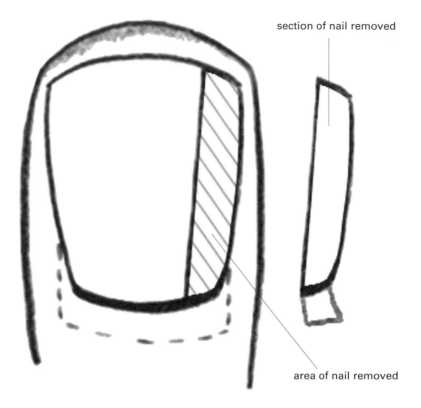

section of nail removed

area of nail removed

Figure 3-2 Removing nail wedge for avulsion or matrixectomy.

Total nail avulsion with a partial matrixectomy
- This is the last option. The entire nail is removed, but only the side of the nail (where the nail is ingrown) is killed with the chemical. This central nail will regrow. I recommend this for patients with fungal nails. This will allow treatment of the fungal nail as it regrows. Another option is to remove the entire nail permanently.

Soaking is advised with any of the treatments. This involves warm water and epsom salt, or the use of a small amount of betadine instead of the epsom salt. Soak the feet for 15 to 20 minutes.

Injections

Injecting the toe to numb it is necessary for nail avulsions and matrixectomies. I give injections almost everyday, to different types of people. I have yet to hear someone say that they enjoy or like needles. Some patients do ask for injections, but only because they are in so much pain. I have many patient encounters that involve injections and high anxiety. I have found that, in general, the most relaxed patients have the least amount of pain.

Toenail removals are a very common procedure for the podiatrist. Many patients are quite anxious before they have the procedure. No one seems to know what to expect. Most people are worried the about the injection. "Will it hurt?" "How long will it take?" "How long is the needle?" "Is it like a bee-sting?"

I try to avoid questioning like this. I have found that the more people focus on the injection and how badly it will hurt, the more it will hurt.

Am I implying that pain is all in your head? Yes and No. Pain is transmitted from your body to your brain via long nerves in the back, so yes in this sense, it is in your head. But is it psychological? Yes and no. Yes in the sense that there are certain factors that can decrease your pain threshold. I have found that when patients

Just Relax

During the day seeing patients, I proceeded into a room with one of my patients in the chair. She was scheduled to have her toenail removed, and was quite nervous about the injection. She squirmed in the chair and thought about changing the date of the procedure. Finally, she said "Ok, let's do it and get it over with." I proceeded as usual. She said "I just need a minute to meditate and then I'll be focused on my breathing." I gladly gave her a minute and then gave her the injection. Not only did she not move during the injection, I don't believe her breathing changed either. And I am quite certain that her breathing was much slower than mine. When I was finished, she took a minute and then said "I didn't feel a thing, you're good!" I smiled "No, it's you who's good."

One day I entered the room to do an injection on a patient of mine who was quite anxious. He asked all of the usual questions ... twice. I answered patiently as he thought of at least 10 more minutes of questions that delayed the injection. I finally convinced him it was time for the injection. He tossed and turned and squirmed. No matter how much anesthetic I put in, he just wouldn't become numb. I gave up after injecting with 3-4 times the normal amount of anesthetic I use to numb a patient's toe. I told him we'd have to do it another day.

I couldn't find a logical reason why he didn't become numb after all of the anesthetic. Technically and medically speaking it seemed impossible. But was it? I gave him one pill to take before his next visit to relax him, and told him to come relaxed for the next visit. He then confessed to having an extremely stressful day at work.

When he returned in two days, he came in before work and had taken the pill to relax him. His wife accompanied him for support. On this day, I used less than the normal amount of anesthetic to completely numb his toe, the procedure was very successful and he didn't have any pain.

are stressed and anxious about procedures or injections they experience more pain. The same injection on a relaxed person appears to be much less painful. Specific pain thresholds can vary. It is my experience that patients who read or talk, or meditate, or do deep breathing usually have less pain during an injection than other patients. When patients are distracted, they are not as focused on the pain. The patients who ask about the time it takes to complete the procedure, ask about the amount and type of pain, and watch the procedure, usually experience more pain.

When people are stressed, their pain threshold appears to decrease, and they experience more pain. The longer the period a patient is exposed to a pain stimulus (like a needle) the greater pain they appear to experience. It is common for people to say "I just can't take it anymore!" And this is true. The same thing that caused them minimal pain 10 minutes ago, may cause them more pain at the present time.

Pain from injections is also decreased by using another

stimulus. For example, a cold spray can be used with injections. This cold spray is applied first. It is very cold, and numbs the skin, but also acts as a counter-irritant. This means that it is trying to fool your brain by causing two different sensations at the same time, in hope that the brain will only process the first one.

"Why can't you numb the toe or the foot before the injection? The dentist does." This is a question I hear at least once a week. It's quite logical to think that the numbing medication the dentist places in your mouth should be effective on other areas of the body. Unfortunately, the only medications that will numb the toe comes out of a needle. The topicals that the dentist uses work very effectively on the mucous membranes such as the lip and the mouth. The tough skin layers, especially on the feet and the hands, will not allow penetration of these topical anesthetics. There are a few creams that can be placed on the skin an hour or two before the injection. They can help numb the skin, but these creams are expensive and usually don't take away all of the pain. You may want to ask your physician about a cream if you feel anxious. If you are very anxious some doctors may prescribe medications to relax you before the procedure. The best way to endure an injection is to relax and not focus on the pain.

The Bottom Line

If you have had an ingrown nail only once, and you remember that it occurred after a specific event, activity or when wearing certain shoes, then the nail avulsion is your best option. If you have had problems with chronic ingrown nails, then the matrixectomy is your best option.

Those Aching Feet

Foot Fungus

tin·e·a pe·dis

Overview

Tinea pedis, or foot fungus, is a common foot ailment. It is caused by fungus invading the foot through small breaks in the skin. As previously discussed with nail fungus, some individuals are naturally susceptible to foot fungus. Those individuals with diabetes and those on *immunosuppresive* medications, such as prednisone, are also more susceptible. As we age, our collagen bonds in the skin are not as strong. As they become weaker, certain things, such as increased moisture and microtrauma can allow for small breaks in the skin and allow for the fungus to invade.

What You See and Feel

The most common symptoms of foot fungus are peeling and itching, with some redness on the bottom of both of the feet. This can range from a mild infection, just at the front of the foot, to a severe infection, encompassing the entire foot (described as a moccasin distribution). The fungus can cause itching, burning, pain or tingling. It can also occur between the toes (*interdigital tinea*) and usually looks like peeling with surrounding white tissue between the toes. The fungus can also appear as patchy red areas on the top of the feet, and sometimes may also appear in circular patterns. Sometimes, the fungus can cause tiny blisters at the bottom of the feet, or in between the toes (*vesicular tinea*).

How To Diagnosis It

Again, usually the diagnosis is purely a clinical evaluation. Skin scrappings can be used for a *KOH* (as described in the Chapter 3) or for a fungal culture, but this is not usually necessary.

What Else Could It Be?

It could be a dermatitis. This can look like a fungus as a patchy red peeling area on the top or bottom of the feet. *Erythrasma* is an infection that also looks like the fungus and occurs between the toes. Erythrasma is fairly uncommon. A bacterial infection can occur in association with a fungus and make the fungus look more like a common infection. This can sometimes make your diagnosis more difficult. Sometimes the dry flakey skin is just that...dry, flakey skin.

What You Can Do About It

The most common treatment is to use a topical anti-fungal medication. Many of the over-the-counter medications work very well, for instance Lamisil®, Lotrimin®, Desenex®, or Tinactin®. I recommend a cream for the feet and a powder or spray for between the toes. Do not put cream between the toes. If these do not work, there are prescription creams that are stronger that you can obtain from your physician. If there is a lot of inflammation, a topical steroid like hydrocortisone can be added. Use the cream for two to

- If you go to the gym, make sure you wear shoes or sandals in the locker room and the shower. This is where foot fungus loves to hang out.
- Bleach out your shower weekly while you are using the medication. Your shower is also another place that fungus likes to hide.
- Put anti-fungal powder in your shoes everyday and let them air out. Your shoes harbor fungus as well.
- Make sure you change your socks once a day, more if you sweat a lot. Never re-wear a pair of socks without washing them first.
- For severe cases, consider using an anti-fungal powder with a carpet freshener on the carpet. Vacuum this up after it sits for an hour. Do this once a month.
- Fungus can be picked up by other family members who use your shower.

four weeks once a day or twice a day depending on the instructions.

Feet that sweat excessively (hyperhydrosis) should be bathed daily in luke warm water and astringent. Using Burrows® soaks 1:40 dilution may be helpful. Dry the feet and place talcum powder or tannic acid powder on, to reduce further sweating. Excess sweating can change the pH of the surface of the skin. This can make it easier for the fungus to thrive in the environment; for instance in a sock or a shoe. Some find using an antiperspirant spray helpful. A roll-on will also work to help decrease moisture on the feet.

The most common reason patients do not get better using topical therapy is because of reinfection. Patients will start to get better because they are using the cream, but end up getting infected again. Common places that cause re-infection are the gym, the shower and a patient's own shoes. To help avoid reinfection, bleach out your shower or tub once or twice a week and put anti-fungal powder in your shoes after you wear them.

The last resort for treatment is oral anti-fungal therapy. These medication are taken in short courses, usually for one week. They are the same medications mentioned in the chapter on fungal nails. The side effects with taking them for seven days are minimal. Most foot fungal infections of the skin can be relieved without taking oral anti-fungal medication.

The Bottom Line

Start with the over the counter topical creams and use them everyday, twice a day, or as instructed. Take precautions to avoid reinfection. If in two to four weeks, the infection is not better, than see your physician. You may receive a prescription anti-fungal medication. If one to two months of diligent application doesn't relieve the redness, itching and peeling, you may want to take a short course of oral medication.

Warts

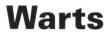

ver•ru•cae

Overview

Warts (also known as *verrucae)* are caused by a virus. Some individuals have an inherited tendency to develop warts. The virus can also be implanted into the skin by a splinter or a piece of glass. Even chronic pressure can drive the virus into the skin. When there are small cuts or breaks in the skin (this can happen with increased water exposure) the virus can invade. Warts are commonly picked up at the gym. Children and people with weakened immune systems can be more vulnerable to the virus. Warts have their own blood and nerve supply which makes them bleed periodically and often very painful.

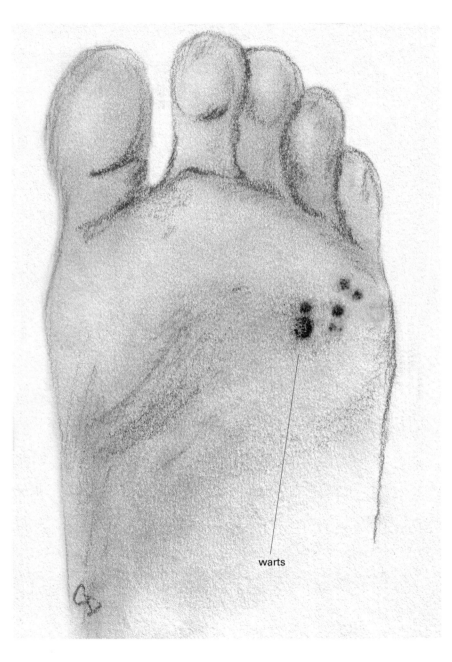

warts

Figure 5-1 warts on the bottom of the foot

Those Aching Feet

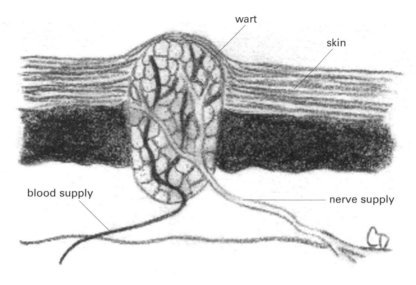

Figure 5-2 blood and nerve supply to the wart

What You See and Feel

Most people notice warts only after they have been there for a while. As it develops it usually looks like a *callous*, but progressively gets worse and become more and more painful. Some warts look like small translucent dots that occur in small groups or clusters. Other warts are large and covered with callous tissue. With trimming, they have pinpoint black areas and may have string-like attachments to the underlying skin. Small lucent areas can be at the center. They are very tender when squeezed and less so when pushed on. When they are *debrided* by a physician, many times there is pinpoint bleeding.

How It's Diagnosed

Once the surrounding callous tissue has been scrapped away an accurate diagnosis can be made. The wart will appear as the description above and will be painful when squeezed. The top layer of skin should be removed (debrided) in order to fully evaluate the lesion.

What Else Could It Be?

A callous is the most common misdiagnosis made when evaluating a wart. It commonly appears exactly like a wart, and that is why it is necessary to remove the top layer of skin when making the diagnosis. Other common misdiagnosis can be a foreign object, for instance a splinter or a piece of glass. Many times this is initially the cause of discomfort. Once the foreign object is removed, the pain continues because a wart has developed.

What You Can Do

There are many treatments for warts. Some of the treatments you can do yourself, others you need to see your physician regularly for. This is not a complete list of treatments, but it will give you an idea of the most common treatments.

Over-the-counter treatments
The over the counter treatments can be effective for a small number of individuals. Make sure not to use the over the counter wart medication if you are diabetic. The acid may burn the surrounding skin. Also be careful using these in children. Although children respond the best to the over the counter products, they need to be used consistently and can sometimes burn other areas of the skin. Most of the wart treatments in the stores have similar ingredients. Usually the active ingredient is 17% salicylic acid solution

Liquid Nitrogen
Liquid nitrogen is probably the most common treatment you'll receive at your doctor's office. This works very well on the hands, but the warts on the feet seem to be more resistant to this therapy.

Acid treatments
There are different types of acid treatments that are available and commonly used by physicians. Salicylic acid can be used by your doctor and is a 60% concen-

One day I encountered a patient that had seen several different doctors and tried every different therapy for warts for over five years. He had tried acid treatments, liquid nitrogen, laser treatments, surgery and all of the over-the-counter products. He had over one hundred warts clustered on his heel to form what looked like one large wart about three inches round. He limped because of the pain.

After I joined the ranks of the doctors failing to remove the wart with acid treatments or surgery, I turned to a different treatment. I placed him on Tagamet® in high doses and started a treatment called "needling". It is a painful treatment, involving multiple injections every two weeks. At first, it only caused him pain, but after 6 weeks he started to notice a difference.

Within an eight month period the warts were completely gone. Fortunately, his case is rare, and not many will have to undergo this form of aggressive therapy. At his last office visit, there were still no signs of the warts one year after starting the treatment.

tration. The salicylic acid is used under occlusion (under a non-breathable bandage) for three to five days for it to be the most effective.

Trichloracetic acid and Canthacur®
Trichloracetic acid can also be used, separately, or in combination with salicylic acid. Another topical treatment is Canthacur®. It is applied weekly at the doctor's office.

Aldara®
A prescription medication for warts. Aldara® is to be applied 3-4 times each week at home.

Hyphercator and 5-flourouracil
Other therapies include the hyphercator, an electric current, and cremes like 5-flourouracil, but these are not commonly used.

Surgical treatment
Surgery involves numbing the area and then excising the lesion. A blade, laser or cautery is used. The surgery usually involves three weeks for the tissue to fill in and

heal and even after the surgical removal there is a chance of recurrence.

Controversial therapies - Needling

Some controversial therapies included needling and oral medications. Needling involves numbing the area and using a needle to penetrate deep into the skin 100 to 200 times. This can be a very painful therapy and is only used in very resistant cases.

Controversial therapies - Oral therapy

Cimetidine, or Tagamet®, which is commonly taken to help stomach ulcers, is also a controversial treatment. Taken in higher doses, Cimetidine has been postulated to boost the immune system. High doses of vitamin A is another controversial option. These therapies have had a mixed response from physicians. Although I have been able make resistant warts disappear with these therapies, I only use these methods in severe cases that are not responsive to any other treatments.

Unfortunately, with all of the treatments mentioned, the warts can still return. The treatments are very individual and people respond differently.

The Bottom Line

There are many treatments for warts. They are extremely difficult to remove. They always have a chance of coming back whether they are surgically removed or removed by acid treatments. They may take one treatment or they may take 50 treatments. Usually, the longer they are there, the harder they will be to resolve. Be sure to see a doctor as soon as you realize that you have a wart.

Do not try cimetidine therapy or vitamin A therapy without consulting a physician.

The key to wart treatment: **act fast!**

Corns and Callouses

hy·per·ker·a·to·sis

Overview

Corns and *callouses* are really just dead skin built up over an area of pressure. *Hyperkeratosis* is the medical term for the build up of that dead skin. Corns and callouses are actually bone problems and not skin problems. When a joint is contracted (in a crooked position) or a bone spur causes increased rubbing on the shoe or the ground, the body will build up *hyperkeratotic tissue* (dead tissue) to protect itself. This dead tissue is callous tissue. If the body does not create the dead tissue, then there is a chance that the skin will wear down and cause an *ulcer* (an opening in the skin).

A corn is usually on the top of a toe, or in-between a toe, whereas a callous is usually on the bottom of the foot or on the heel. Both can be extremely painful if

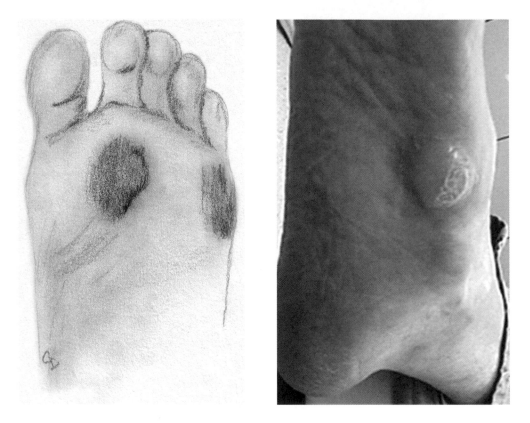

Figure 6-1 callous formation

they become large. If they become large then the pressure from the ground or the shoe causes pain. Typically the corn on the top of the toe is only painful when the shoe rubs the toe.

The fifth toe (small toe) commonly has a corn on the side. This is usually due to the toe turning in (*adducto-varus*) or having only one joint instead of two. This leads to a greater chance of developing a corn on the 5th toe. This occurs in about 40% of the population.

What You See and Feel

A corn is usually a small amount of thickened skin at the area of a joint on top of one of the toes. Usually the toe is a *hammertoe*. It can also be at the side of a toe due to a bone spur. Corns can also appear as soft tissue between the toes, this is also called a soft corn or a web corn. Most of these occur between the 4th and the 5th toe. These build up because the joints are rubbing on each other. Sometimes they appear white and sometimes they can have a core (deep area of skin build-up in the center).

A callous is usually broader, and occurs under the ball of the foot, under the joints. Callouses also can have a core, or a central area that is deep and painful. The callouses usually build up quickly. Other areas are the sides of the big toe and the inside or outside of the heel. When callouses build up at the side of the toe, and the heel, then usually the problem is due to abnormal movement of the foot, which is outlined in Chapter 11 on *flatfeet*.

How It's Diagnosed

There is little clinical observation that needs to be made to diagnose a corn or a callous. Where the physician

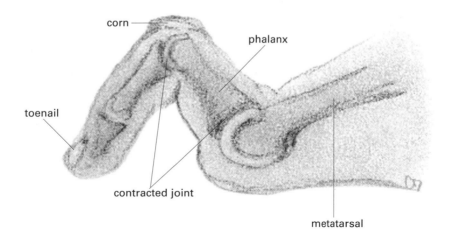

Figure 6-2 hammertoe with corn

makes a difference, especially your podiatrist, is the ability to tell you why it is forming. A hammertoe causing a corn is fairly obvious. Most corns between the toes or callouses on the bottom of the feet are caused by biomechanical problems. In order to find out why these callouses are building up, an individual needs to be seen by a physician trained in biomechanics. As I mentioned earlier, many callouses are due to abnormal motion. *Pronation* (the feet rolling in) is a common cause of callouses. Sometimes the great toe joint does not take it's fair share of the weight, and hence the 2nd toe joint becomes overloaded and a painful callouses develops. There are many different types of feet, and many different types of callous patterns.

What Else Could It Be?

The most common mis-diagnosis for a callous is a wart. This is a common mistake because they can look quite similar. Fortunately, wart treatments, although they will not "cure" the callous, they will not hurt the callous.

What You Can Do About It

Treating a callous or a corn is a two step process.

Step One: Remove dead tissue build-up and decrease pressure.
- There are corn and callous medicated pads at the drug store. I do not recommend these.
- These usually will not take away the corn and may cause a chemical burn of the surrounding skin.
- Your physician may remove the build-up of tissue with a sharp blade. This is not surgery, this is only removing the dead skin.
- Donut hole pads that tend to take pressure off the area are an effective form of treatment. These will allow the pressure of the shoe or the ground to be dispersed to other areas of the foot and not on the corn or callous.
- Using a pumice stone to keep the dead tissue from building up is also another form of therapy. (Pumice

Avoid medicated pads if you are diabetic.

stones are not recommended for diabetics)
- There are creams available that help decrease callous tissue. Some examples are Kerasal®, and urea cream. They may be difficult to find in a pharmacy and may need a prescription. I suggest asking your physician.

Step Two: Go after the problem.
- This means trying to find the reason you are getting the callous and then fixing this problem.
- A callous or corn can not just be cut out. Since it is a bone problem, cutting it out will only be temporary relief, it will eventually return.
- If the corn is there because of a hammertoe, the treatment of choice is to find shoes that don't rub on your toe, use pads to keep the pressure off the toe, or use a buttress pad to straighten the toe. If these don't help then you may need surgery.
- If the callous exists because of abnormal motion in your foot, then orthotics will help control that motion and decrease the build up of the dead tissue.
- If you have a bunion (see chapter 9) and that is causing a callous, you may need surgery on the bunion in order to have the callous disappear.

The Bottom Line

If you have callouses, first try daily treatments with lotions and a pumice stone. Stop wearing shoes that are too tight, or may cause rubbing. If the condition still persists, see a podiatrist. A podiatrist is very knowledgeable about foot biomechanics and can help you with your treatment decisions.

7

Hammertoes

Overview

Hammertoes are usually a result of tendon imbalance and/or abnormal motion in the foot. Most people who have hammertoes have an abnormal shape to their foot (high arch or low arch) or have some abnormal motion that results in the tendons pulling the toes up. Shoes can cause irritation and callous build-up resulting in pain. A full evaluation by a physician knowledgeable in *biomechanics* of the foot is needed to truly determine the *etiology* or cause.

What You See and Feel

The toes are pulled up by the tendons on the top of the foot, and the tips of the toes are crooked and curled down. Sometimes the top of the toes or the tips of the toes develop corns. Hammertoes can be very painful or

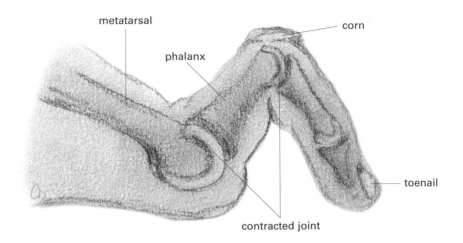

metatarsal

corn

phalanx

toenail

contracted joint

Figure 7-1 hammertoe with corn

they may not hurt at all. Some toes are very flexible and some are very rigid. The rigid hammertoes are usually quite painful. Pain usually occurs when the patient wears shoes, whether they are idle or walking.

How It's Diagnosed

Diagnosis is much more than looking at a crooked, curled toe and calling it a "hammertoe." The difficulty in the diagnosis is determining why you have hammertoes. X-rays are taken to see the position of the bones. There may be a small or large curl (contracture) of the toe. An exam of the entire foot is necessary. This helps the doctor determine why the hammertoes developed.

What You Can Do About It

The type of treatment you choose depends upon the cause and the type of your hammertoe. There are two types of hammertoes, flexible and rigid.

Flexible Hammertoes
If the hammertoe is only moderately painful and the hammertoe is flexible, many individuals can get full relief from padding and *debridements* (callous removal).

Those Aching Feet

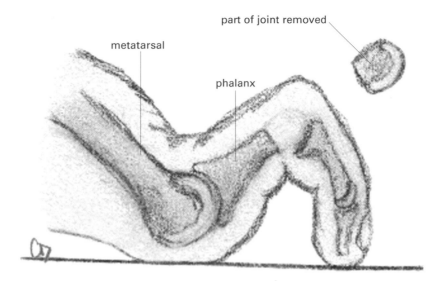

metatarsal

part of joint removed

phalanx

Figure 7-2 removing joint during surgery

Donut hole pads purchased at the local drug store can be placed on top of the toe and help relieve pressure and pain. Buttress pads made by your podiatrist can help straighten out the toes and prevent the callous formation that causes painful corns. Buttress pads may also be purchased at the store or in speciality catalogs. Wide shoes can help decrease pressure, and therefore decrease callous buildup which will decrease pain.

Rigid Hammertoes

If your hammertoes still curl under when you stand, or when your doctor pushes down on them, then they are rigid. Conservative treatments will usually not work very well. Certain types of padding as well as wider shoes should be tried, and can relieve pain for a number of years. Surgical treatment is the next step.

What You Can Do About It: Surgery

The common surgeries for a hammertoe are called an *arthroplasty* or *arthrodesis*. An arthroplasty is the removal of the joint that is causing the pressure. The arthroplasty may involve releasing the ligaments at the joint in the foot and may also require a pin placed in the bone. Sometimes the ligaments at the base of the toe need to be cut and loosened. After surgery, walking in a post-surgical shoe for a minimum of two weeks is required.

An arthrodesis is the fusing of the joint (placing the two bones together so that there is no movement). Fusing the joint usually requires releasing the ligaments and putting a pin in the toe. This requires four to six weeks in the surgical shoe depending on how long the pin is in. The pin is removed in the office.

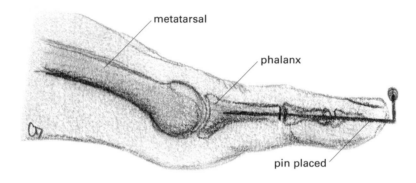

metatarsal

phalanx

pin placed

Figure 7-3 straightened toe with pin placed after surgery

Both of these procedures involve a 30 minute surgery which can be done at the office, hospital or at a surgery center. (Time spent at the hospital or surgery center is usually much longer.)

The toes can remain swollen for many weeks after the surgery. In general, swelling is very difficult to get out of the toes.

A few reasons for prolonged swelling are listed below:
• The toes are the furthest from the heart.

- There is no pumping mechanism at that level. (When the muscles in the legs contract, they press on the veins and help to pump the blood back to the heart.)
- Gravity is a large factor as well, and as we all know, we spend many hours a day on our feet.
- All of these factors contribute to prolonged swelling after any surgery of the feet and especially after surgery of the toe.

The Bottom Line

Always try conservative treatment first and consider surgery as a last resort. For the diabetic who has no feeling in the feet, a potential *ulceration* is a serious consequence. Surgical repair is necessary if the blood flow is adequate.

8

Bunions

hal·lux ab·duc·to val·gus

Overview

A *bunion* is a bone deformity at the great toe joint. The
1st *metatarsal* (long bone at the inside of the foot) moves
towards the center of the body (*medial*) and the big toe
moves towards the small toes (*lateral*). (See Figure 8-1)
This movement causes a large bump at the inside of the
foot. This is rarely a bone growth. This bump is usually
a result of abnormal motion (usually *pronation*). The
tendons can also contribute to the deformity as well.

What You See and Feel

The great toe joint will usually drift to the side and
cause a bump long before the pain develops. This is
usually a slow process and takes a few years to
develop. Pain and/or callous usually develops next,

and that is when most people ask their physician for treatment options. The pain is usually dull and occurs with walking and shoe pressure. Sometimes in the advanced stages, when arthritis sets in, there can be a grinding feeling, sharp pain and limited motion. Throbbing can occur while sitting, standing or walking without shoes.

How It's Diagnosed

The diagnosis of a bunion can be made by any physician, but the stage that the bunion is in, needs to be evaluated by a foot specialist. Your physician will press on the toe to see where most of the pain is. He or she will also move it up and down. The more advanced the bunion, the more pain the patient will have with pressure and with movement. Some individuals do not experience pain with movement of the toe. If there is grinding with movement, or little or no movement at all, then the bunion is in an advanced stage.

Some bunions press up against the 2nd toe and can cause pain. They can also cause the 2nd toe to pop up and sit on top of the great toe. These are also signs of an advanced stage. If there is a lot of pain or surgery is considered, then x-rays will be taken. This will allow the physician to evaluate the bone structure, the overall structure of the foot, as well the condition of the joint.

Oh, That Old Bunion

An 85 year old woman came to my office complaining of foot pain. She gave no indication of where the pain was on her "patient information" form. When I saw her large bunion, I automatically assumed that was her foot pain. I spent the first few minutes questioning her about the pain, and looking at a very severe bunion deformity. When her pain complaints didn't correlate to a bunion, I asked her to point to her pain. She then pointed to her 5th toe. Confused, I pointed to the bunion. "Do you have any pain here?" She replied "Oh, that old thing. Nah...it just makes it hard to find shoes. I don't have any pain there, but that little toe, it is just killing me!"

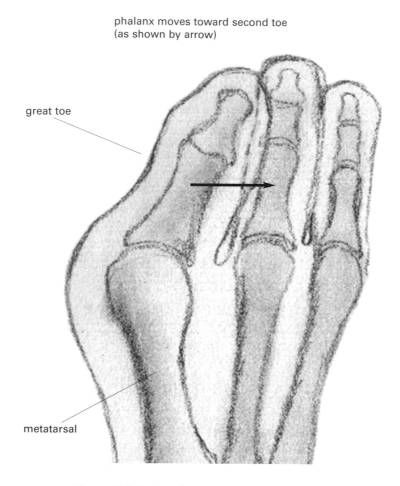

phalanx moves toward second toe
(as shown by arrow)

great toe

metatarsal

Figure 8-1 bunion: first metatarsal moves towards inside of foot
and great toe moves towards outside of foot

What Else Could It Be?

There are not many other problems that appear like a
bunion. Some joints that have arthritis and don't move
well may appear to be bunions. A large bursa (protective fluid sac) can form and make the bunion appear
more severe. Gout can occur at this joint and appear
like a bunion. Gout is much more painful and red than
the typical bunion. When there is a bump on top of the
foot, instead of on the side of the foot, it is called a dorsal bunion. The treatment for this is slightly different
from the treatment for a regular bunion.

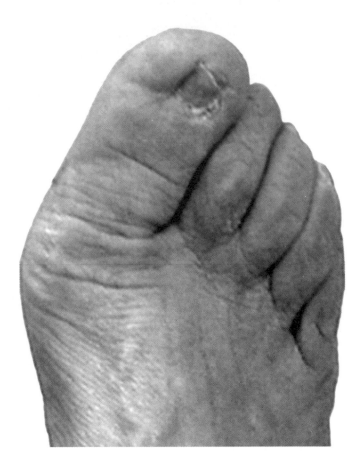

Figure 8-2 bunion deformity, right foot

What You Can Do About It

Unfortunately, there are only a few conservative treatments for bunions. Here are some things you can try.

Pads and wider shoes
If the symptoms are minimal then using pads on the bump and wearing wider shoes can give a lot of relief.

Orthotics
Orthotics may give some relief and may slow progression of the deformity. As with many other foot deformities, abnormal pronation can indirectly cause bunions. Orthotics will help keep the foot in a normal

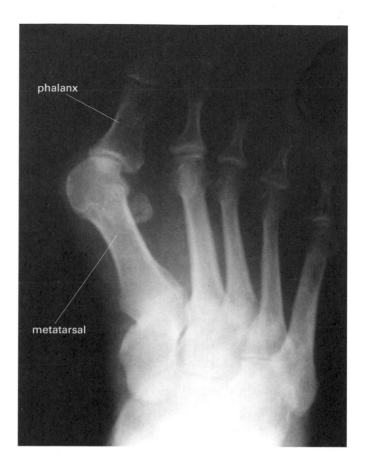

phalanx

metatarsal

Figure 8-3 x-ray of a bunion deformity, right foot

position and attempt to eliminate the abnormal motion.

Bunion night splints
Bunion night splints will usually not change the deformity. Some patients feel that the night splints help reduce any pain that occurs as a result of pressure while sleeping. Keep in mind that this is a bone problem, not a soft tissue problem. The night splint will not correct a bone problem.

Anti-inflammatory medication (NSAID)
Anti-inflammatory medication, like ibuprofen, can help to decrease pain by decreasing inflammation. Anti-inflammatory medication is commonly termed

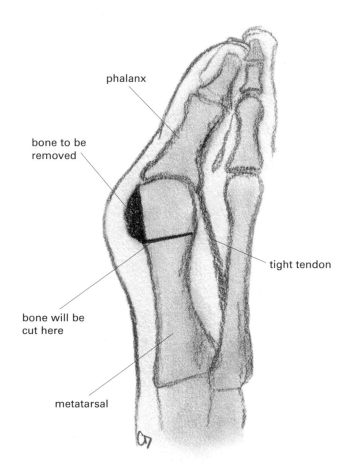

phalanx

bone to be removed

bone will be cut here

tight tendon

metatarsal

Figure 8-4 bunion surgery outlined

NSAIDS. NSAIDS stands for **N**on **S**teroidal **A**nti-**I**nflammatory **D**rugs. This class of drugs includes Motrin®, Advil®, Relafen®, Daypro®, Naprosyn®, Feldene®, aspirin and many others. Tylenol® (acetaminophen) is not an anti-inflammatory drug. COX-2 inhibitors, like Vioxx® and Celebrex® are the most common NSAIDS, and they are easier on the stomach.

Contrast soaks
Another form of therapy is contrast soaks. Use alternating hot and cold soaks or you can alternate between hot and cold packs. First place an ice pack on your foot, then switch to a warm pack and finally return to the ice pack. Switch back and forth, using each pack in 5 min-

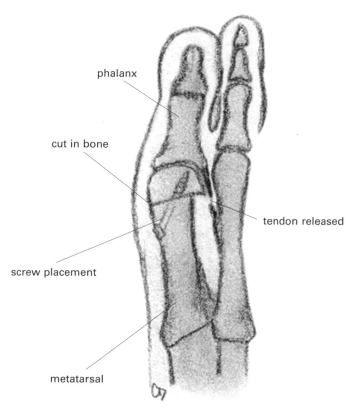

phalanx

cut in bone

tendon released

screw placement

metatarsal

Figure 8-5 bunion surgery performed

COX-2 Inhibitors

There has been quite a bit of controversy surrounding NSAIDS, especially the COX-II inhibitors. Vioxx was taken off the market in late 2004 due to concerns of increased adverse cardiovascular events, which includes heart attacks and stroke. Other COX-II inhibitors, such as Celebrex® and Bextra®, are similarly under fire. Even Naproxen, a widely used NSAID, available since 1976, has been linked to cardiovascular deaths.

What does this all mean? Who and which study do you believe? As of January 2005, there is no common consensus about which NSAIDS are not safe. Some experts feel COX-II inhibitors have been over-prescribed without justifiable indication. Others feel that the studies tell us nothing about the risk for individuals under 70 years of age taking NSAIDS for short periods of time.

Even if you do not have increased risk for GI complications (bleeding, gastritis, GERD), or an increased risk for heart disease, you should talk with your physician about risks and benefits of such drugs based on your personal health history.

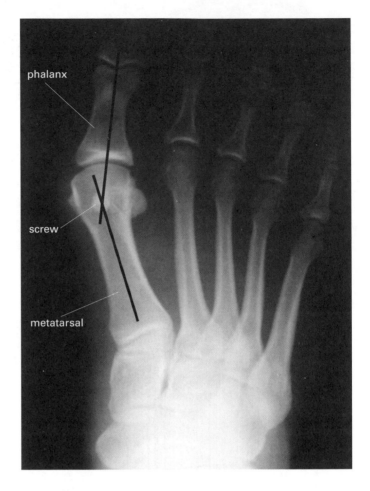

phalanx

screw

metatarsal

Figure 8-6 x-ray before bunion surgery

utes intervals, for a total of 30 minutes. Ice for 5 minutes, warm for 5 minutes, ice for 5 minutes, and repeat.

Ice pack
Use an ice pack at the end of the day for 20 minutes. Do not place ice directly on foot. Use a pack, or place a towel between the ice and your skin.

Range of motion exercises
This involves moving the toe up, holding it for 20 seconds and then moving it down and holding it for 20 seconds. Do about five sets, twice a day. It will help if

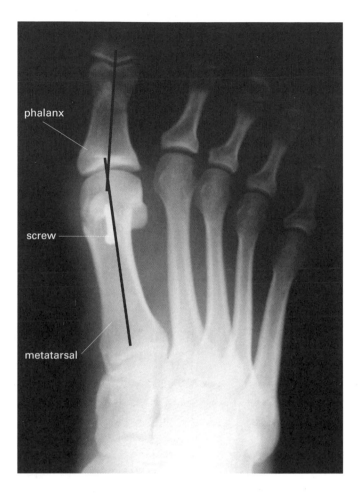

phalanx

screw

metatarsal

Figure 8-7 x-ray after bunionectomy

you soak your foot in warm water for 20 minutes before you start motion exercises. This will help to loosen up the ligaments.

Stop walking up hills
This may significantly decrease the pain. Excess stress goes through the big toe joint when going up hills.

Rockerbottom shoe or roll bar
If the joint is limited in movement, then a rockerbottom shoe, or roll bar in a shoe may help.

Chondroitin sulfate and glucosamine

These are two supplements that are available at your local drug store. A prescription is not needed. Studies dating back to the 1980's show signs that these two supplements can help relieve the pain of arthritis. These supplements are postulated to enhance the cartilage at a biochemical level. The typical dose of these supplements varies and is usually listed on the label. It is recommended to take 1,000 mg to 2,000 mg of glucosamine and 800 mg to 1,600 mg of chondroitin sulfate a day. If you can tolerate some medical terminology, I highly recommend *The Arthritis Cure* by Jason Theodosakis, M.D., Brenda Adderly, M.H.A. and Barry Fox, Ph.D. This book describes arthritis, it's causes, new approaches to treatments and discusses in detail the use of glucosamine and chondroitin sulfate.

What You Can Do About It: Surgery Options

When the bunion is causing a lot of pain or there is a lot of arthritis associated with the joint, then surgery is recommended. There are various types of surgery that correct the deformity. The most common surgery involves breaking the bone in the foot, the metatarsal, near the toe and placing a pin, a screw or a staple in the bone (See Figures 8-4 and 8-5). After surgery, a surgical shoe must be worn for six weeks. Sometimes surgeons will place patients in regular shoes at three to four weeks if a screw or other form of stable fixation is used. Bone takes six weeks to heal, and return to regular walking activities usually occurs at six to eight weeks. Figure 8-6 shows an x-ray of a mild, but painful bunion. Figure 8-7 shows the bunion after surgery. Although the correction may seem subtle, note the difference in spacing between the first and second toes.

Some bunions require more advanced surgery. Breaks in the bone are made towards the middle of the foot, and sometimes fusion of a joint is necessary. Tendon lengthenings and transfers may also be necessary. In

Be Skeptical
If your doctor says that you will be in a regular shoe one weeks after surgery, get a second opinion. He or she may not be doing the correct procedure.

order to know which procedure is the best for you, a full evaluation by a podiatric surgeon or an orthopedic surgeon who does foot surgery is necessary. The post-operative course is usually much longer with these advanced procedures and may involve a cast requiring no weight on the foot and the use of crutches for two months.

The Bottom Line

You don't have pain? .....don't have surgery.

Useful tips to help with your decision:

- If you only have a small deformity and don't have much pain, the pain may be relieved by a change in shoes, a change in walking habits and taking anti-inflammatory medications.
- If you have pain everyday that is getting in the way or your daily activities, then it may be time for you to consider surgery.
- If you have diabetes with some loss of nerve sensation in your feet and have good blood supply, I recommend having surgery on your bunion if it is causing callouses and pain.
- If you have a significant deformity with only mild pain, take into consideration that the joint will eventually deteriorate and develop arthritis. Once you have arthritis, surgery will not correct the arthritis, only the deformity.

9

Heel Pain

plan·tar fas·ci·i·tis

Overview

Heel pain is one of the most common problems that a podiatrist sees. The most common diagnosis for heel pain is *plantar fasciitis*. Another name commonly heard is "heel spur syndrome." Plantar means bottom of the foot. The *fascia* is a long ligament type structure. "Itis" means inflammation. Plantar fasciitis is tearing and inflammation of the long ligament on the bottom of the foot. This is a result of small micro-tears in the fascia due to overstress. A spur can develop as a result of the pull and stress of the fascia on the bone, but it is rarely the cause of pain. Many people may think that the pain is due to the bone spur, but very few bone spurs cause pain. In fact, many individuals with bone spurs do not have any pain at all. Only 50% of those individuals with plantar fasciitis have a heel spur. Most of the time the heel spur does not cause the pain.

Snowball Effect
small tears
↓
inflammation
↓
fascia is weakened
↓
more walking
↓
more tearing
↓
more inflammation
↓
more tearing

So why do we get heel pain? Most people have abnormal motion in their feet, usually pronation. When the feet turn in and collapse, the fascia takes on an extra stress at the heel. It only takes a small change in activity or change in shoes to cause a small tear, if you are prone to this condition. People who are prone to this condition, usually have low arch feet. Individuals with high arch feet can have fasciitis as well. The tearing that occurs at the fascia, near the heel, is microscopic. This is not a full rupture. But it is enough to weaken the fascia. Once it is weakened, it tears more, then it becomes more inflamed, then it tears more. I call it the "snowball effect". The constant weight of the body on the feet puts a tremendous force load through the feet. When the foot is injured, the injury becomes worse with each step. The average person takes approximately 8,000 to 10,000 steps in a day, so you can imagine how a small tear can develop into a big problem.

What You See and Feel

The most common symptom of plantar fasciitis is sharp pain at the heel, at the first step in the morning or after long periods of rest. This pain usually lessens after 10-15 minutes with walking, but will progressively get worse by the end of the day. Most people notice a gradual increase in pain over many months, but some notice significant development of pain after a few weeks. There is usually no shooting pain to the toes, numbness or tingling associated with the pain. Plantar Fasciitis can be felt in other ways , such as at the end of the day, or only when doing certain sports like running, jogging or walking.

How It's Diagnosed

History is the most important tool for diagnosis of plantar fasciitis. Although not all people have the symptoms described above, the diagnosis usually can be made before examining the patient. On exam, the patient usually has pain with *palpation* (pressing) of the inside of the heel, and sometimes along the inside of

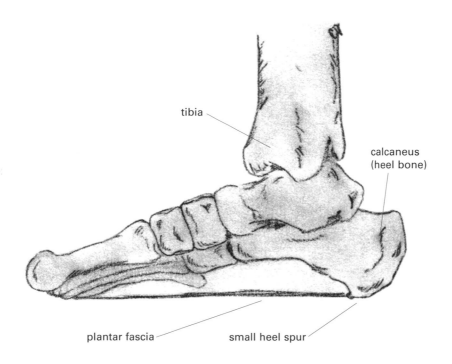

tibia

calcaneus
(heel bone)

plantar fascia

small heel spur

Figure 9-1 plantar fascia and associated heel spur

the arch. These two points are the portions of the fascia under the greatest stress, and these areas have the most pain because they have the most *inflammation* (swelling at a small level).

X-rays are taken to rule out other conditions. Some of these conditions are stress fractures, bone tumors (usually *benign*) and fractures of a heel spur. Although these are usually not common, they do need to be ruled out. Also, the x-ray will allow the doctor to better assess the position of the foot. The x-rays should be taken while standing. A stress fracture of the heel bone, a fracture of the bone spur, or a bone tumor (which is quite uncommon) can be ruled out when an x-ray is taken.

What Else Could It Be?

There are many causes of heel pain. Approximately 90% of people who experience heel pain have plantar fasciitis, or some variation of plantar fasciitis. Other causes of heel pain are listed below.

Heel neuroma
This is an inflamed nerve in the same area. It's usually caused by some aggravating factor, such as an injury.

Heel bursa
A *bursa* is a sac of fluid in the body (usually very small) that is built up by the body to protect it from abnormal pressure. Trauma can cause small ruptures that lead to a bursa formation.

Stress fracture in the heel
A stress *fracture* (broken bone) is not a complete fracture, but a partial fracture. The bone is not completely broken, but over-stressed to a point that there is a very small break within the bone. You could compare a stress fracture to a small crack in a ceramic cup. You know that the cup is cracked, but it is not completely broken. It will still function as a cup and not leak, but it is weakened. This is the same for many bones in the body. A stress fracture does not initially show up on x-ray. Usually a stress fracture doesn't show up on the x-ray for about two to four weeks. In most cases, the stress fracture causes the body to send a lot of blood to the area to heal it. This results in swelling within the heel and results in pain.

Heel spur fracture
Some individuals may have heel spurs and not even know it. Some may over stress their feet by walking too much, or jumping and landing wrong, which can cause a fracture of a spur. This is fairly uncommon and usually results in *acute* (instant) pain, bruising and swelling. An x-ray will show if there is a fracture of the spur.

Plantar Fasciosis?

"Plantar" means bottom, "Fascia" describes the long ligament in the bottom of the foot and "Itis" means inflammation, hence the term plantar fasciitis. Some researchers have looked at the fascia under the microscope and found more evidence of degeneration (breakdown of tissue) than inflammation. "Osis" means abnormal condition and some feel plantar fasci-"itis" would be better termed plantar fasci - "osis". Further research may lead to changes in our current methods of treatment in the future.

Full fracture of the heel (broken heel bone)

It's possible to break your heel bone, but doctors do not confuse it with fasciitis. There is a very sudden onset of pain after an injury. Interestingly, the most common cause of heel bone fractures is falling off of a ladder. Usually blunt trauma causes the fracture. Broken heel bones are easy to diagnose on x-ray, and are rarely confused with plantar fasciitis. The one instance that might cause confusion, is the broken heel that occurs with osteoporosis in individuals with poor sensation. For those individuals with osteoporosis, a broken heel can occur without an injury.

Bone tumor

It is very rare to have a bone tumor in the heel. When it does occur it is usually benign. Many times patients will not have pain with the tumor unless the bone fractures.

Bone spur at the back of the heel

A bone spur at the back of the heel is called retrocalcaneal exostosis. This is rarely confused with plantar fasciitis because pain is usually from the shoe rubbing the back of the heel, as opposed to having pain, when walking, on the bottom of the heel. This problem can be associated with Achilles tendonitis and is discussed in "Chapter 14: Athletes".

Arthritis

There are different types of arthritis that are associated with heel pain. There are also some inflammatory bowel diseases that are associated with the heel. Usually the heel pain associated with arthritis is similar to the heel pain with plantar fasciitis. Usually there is a heel spur associated with the heel pain. Some of these disorders include rheumatoid arthritis, Crohn's disease, psoriatic arthritis, ankylosing spondylitis and Reiter's syndrome. These are not as common as fasciitis, and usually appear with other symptoms such as back pain and stiffness or an irritable bowel.

What You Can Do About It

The treatments for plantar fasciitis are usually conservative. This problem can sometimes take eight to twelve months to resolve. The one treatment that often gives the most benefit is the one that no one seems to be able to do: **Rest**. This involves **staying off your feet**, avoiding walking up hills and climbing stairs. It's the most difficult treatment to do because most of us are on our feet all day, either at work or at home. No matter what your day is like, it usually involves a lot of time on your feet.

The most beneficial treatment is to rest and stay off your feet!

Decrease your heel pain by following the steps below:

1. Decrease your activity level

As suggested above, rest, stay off your feet and decrease your overall activity level. This is difficult to do, but it works!

Keeping the load off of your feet

- Stop running, jogging or walking. Swim or bike instead.
- If you work out on a treadmill, stop! This is the worst activity for your heels.
- Avoid the stairmaster. The stairmaster puts a lot of stress through your arch.
- If you are up and down at work a lot, try to limit it. Get up only once an hour, or just once every 2 hours.
- At home you should avoid going up and down the stairs multiple times. When possible, have someone in your household run up or down the stairs for you.
- Try to avoid steep hills. Stairs are better than hills. Walking up stairs sideways will help take the stress off your feet.
- Do not lift or carry heavy items. This adds to the total amount of force that goes through your feet. This also increases the total impact on your heel.
- Do not lift your kids and carry them. Use a stroller, have them walk, or let your spouse/significant other carry them.
- Don't lift weights. If you do, make sure you are seated.
- The elliptical machine can also aggravate plantar fasciitis. To exercise with this, lower the platform adjustment to it's lowest level.
- Avoid going barefoot.

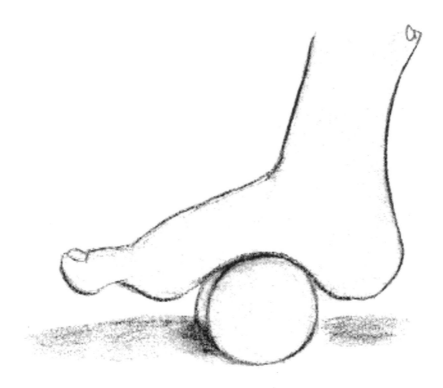

Figure 9-2 ice massage using frozen water bottle

2. Ice massage

Ice massage your heel every day, twice a day, if possible. Freeze a sports water bottle and place it on the floor. Roll your foot over it, in the arch area. (See Figure 9-2) This will stretch out the area and allow the ice to decrease inflammation

3. Stretch your calf muscles (See Figure 9-3)

Most people with plantar fasciitis have tight calf muscles, so stretching can be very beneficial. Do a "runners stretch" by placing your arms against the wall with one leg behind you, straightened and the other leg bent in front. Lean forward, without lifting your heel, until you feel a stretch. This will allow for the calf and fascia to stretch.

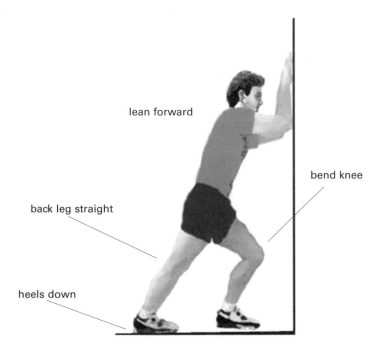

Figure 9-3 calf stretch

Although it seems strange, stretch before getting out of bed, even before putting your feet on the floor. Place a belt or a towel under your forefoot, keep your knee extended, and pull your forefoot towards you, allowing the calf to stretch.

4. Take anti-inflammatory medication

Anti-inflammatory medication like ibuprofen or other NSAIDS will help reduce the pain and inflammation. Take daily for a short period of two to four weeks. You may want to see your doctor for a prescription. Although you can obtain ibuprofen at the local drug store, a prescription from your doctor will be much stronger. Usually taking 600mg to 800mg three times a day is necessary to relieve pain and inflammation. Do not take a dose this high without consulting your doctor. Other medications, similar to ibuprofen, can be beneficial. Discontinue use if you have any stomach problems, bleeding problems or if

Don't take an anti-inflammatory if you currently have a stomach ulcer.

Consult your doctor for alternatives.

you have a history of stomach ulcers.

5. **Heel lifts or heel cups**
   Combined with the above therapies, heel lifts can be very beneficial. When used alone, they provide very little benefit.

6. **Wear good supportive shoes**
   This may seem logical, but most people do not wear supportive shoes. Chapter 11 on flatfeet provides a detailed rundown on how to pick out shoes. It's important to know that the more flexible the shoe, the worse it will be for plantar fasciitis.

7. **Lose Weight**
   This is by far the most frustrating thing someone could tell you! Many of my patients have had the following thoughts or scenarios.

   "How am I going to lose weight when you just told me to stay off of my feet?"

   "My family physician just told me to lose weight. The heel pain began after I started walking to lose weight."

   "I finally decided to lose that extra 20 pounds and when I started running, I developed this heel pain."

   I often encounter patients with these dilemmas. It's very common to encounter heel pain when beginning a new activity. It's also very frustrating to finally decide to lose weight, then develop fasciitis.

Why Your Weight is Important

It is not just your weight that goes through your feet when your heel hits the floor. It is also the speed your leg travels, multiplied by the force of gravity, multiplied by the weight of your leg. When you add more weight to your body (by carrying kids, weight lifting, lifting boxes, or excess body fat) the extra weight isn't just added to the force that goes through your feet, it is multiplied. This is a considerable impact. Also, most active people walk 8,000 to 10,000 steps during a day. Sedentary people walk about 2,000 to 4,000 steps in a day. Small amounts of weight loss and weight gain can significantly affect your feet in the long run.

Get motivated! I suggest that you change your activity. If you have access to a pool, start swimming or doing water aerobics. Walking is the cheapest and easiest form of exercise, and I guarantee that you will be able to do it again. But, for now, you need to alter what you are doing. Leg lifts, sit ups, weight lifting (sitting down only), arm exercises and biking. It is very important to exercise for your health and there are many forms of exercise that don't involve pounding on your feet.

Steps 1-7 are the first steps to treating plantar fasciitis. Doing just one or another by itself will not help reduce your heel pain. You must do all the steps at once to achieve the maximum benefit. I instruct patients to take two weeks out of their busy lives and dedicate this time to these therapies. It may not be right away, but you must be sincere in your attempt at doing the combined therapies or you will be wasting your time.

Other treatments involve steroid injections, orthotics, arch supports, night splints, strappings, soft casts, hard casts, cast boots and crutches. Some people have used contrast soaks, physical therapy, ultrasound and acupuncture with some good results.

If you take the time to do these treatments for just two weeks, you will notice a significant amount of change. I have found that people can have a 50% reduction in pain if they do the therapies properly. After the pain has decreased over the two week period, I usually suggest continuing the therapy for another two weeks, while gradually starting to increase activity. The remaining pain will take a few weeks to a few months to completely go away, but it will be manageable. For a faster recovery period, continue all the therapy diligently until the pain is gone.

Remember, doing these alternative exercises won't last forever.......it's just until your feet have healed.

Are You Really Doing the Therapy?

One of my patients told me that he had been diagnosed with plantar fasciitis two years ago and "not one doctor could make the pain go away". I started to inquire about treatments he had already tried...

"Rest?"...yes
"Anti-inflammatories?" ...yes
"Heel lifts/heel cups?"...yes
"Stretching? Icing?, Physical therapy?"...yes, yes, yes
"Custom orthotics?"....two different pairs
"Steroid injections?"....two

Hmmm! I found out that he was usually quite active, but said he hadn't been able to run in two years. Normally he competed in half marathons. I offered him the more aggressive approach of casting, crutches, injections and PT. He refused any further treatment and said he'd go back to trying the icing and stretching.

That weekend I happened to see him running, at quite a good pace. I questioned him at the next visit about his running. As it turned out, for him, decreasing his activity meant decreasing his running from 50-60 miles a week to 30 miles a week. He also admitted to not taking the anti-inflammatories or icing daily.

I said "I need two weeks from you if you want to improve. Two weeks of absolutely no running. Bike if you must exercise, but no treadmill, jogging, walking or running. Also, I'll do a steroid injection, place you in a cast boot, give you crutches and send you to physical therapy twice a week and you'll do ice therapy every night. You'll need to take anti-inflammatory medications for two weeks...every day."

He reluctantly agreed and followed the regimen carefully. In two weeks he was 80% improved. I started him back walking the first week and then gradually worked him back into running, with a new pair of orthotics and a new pair of shoes. He did experience some pain after returning to running, but it was only about 25% of what it was before. After six weeks he was back to running 50-60 miles again.

The moral: be honest with your doctor. If you haven't done the prescribed therapy, tell her or him. Sometimes taking a few weeks out of your daily routine is enough to get you back on track. His running suffered for two years because he wasn't willing to quit for a few weeks.

What You Can Do About It: See a Doctor

If you feel that you did not benefit from the initial therapy you need to see your doctor for other treatment. Your physician may suggest some of the following:

A steroid injection
This is a very strong anti-inflammatory drug that is injected to the site of inflammation. It is only an anti-inflammatory agent, it will not heal the ligament. I like to think of steroid injections as 'jump starting' the healing process by decreasing inflammation.

Orthotics
Custom made orthotics are devices that are molded specifically to your feet. If your foot has abnormal motion, then orthotics will help keep your foot in the correct position and stop the abnormal motion. Once the abnormal motion has stopped, then the pulling and the tearing of the fascia will be stopped. For certain types of feet with abnormal motion, I always recommend orthotics. This treatment goes directly to the root of the problem and stops the cause of the problem.

Orthotics are not for everyone. Some individuals may have developed fasciitis as an injury and will not benefit from orthotics. Some types of feet don't respond well to orthotics. Instead of pain relief, some people will complain of hip, knee or back pain.

Orthotics can be expensive. If your insurance doesn't cover orthotics, consider trying the conservative therapies first. When you buy an arch support or flexible foot insert at the drug store, you are not buying an orthotic. You are buying something that may help your arch, but will not help control motion. An orthotic helps to control abnormal motion. It is rigid, and hard, but surprisingly comfortable. An arch support will not accomplish this. The best over-the-counter orthotic is a rigid sports orthotic that can be found at a local sports store. I usually recommend Superfeet® orthotics.

Physical therapy

Physical therapy can involve a variety of treatments, including ice baths, contrast soaks, ultrasound, stretching and strengthening. I usually send patients to physical therapy when they have had poor results with the therapies mentioned or if they can't do the recommended home therapy consistently. I have found physical therapy to be time consuming but very effective. Although not everyone has good results with physical therapy, some patients have had great success.

Some home physical therapy includes doing toe curls. Spread a towel out below the feet. Place the feet flat on the towel. Curl toes and drag the towel under the feet. Repeat 10 times, or until there is pain. Stop any therapy if you experience pain.

Night splints

Splints are placed on the feet at night to stretch the calf and the fascia throughout the night. Most studies have shown night splints to be ineffective, but usually this is due to poor patient compliance. This means that the splints are difficult to sleep with. As a result, most people have a difficult time wearing them throughout the night.

Soft casts

This is a cast that is flexible and allows movement, but restricts motion. A soft cast may be helpful when combined with crutches or some of the above mentioned therapies. A soft cast is also referred to as an unna boot.

Hard casts

Hard casts are used in combination with crutches to take all pressure off of the heel, allowing time for healing. They are used only in very severe cases that are resistant to all other therapies. Usually casting and crutches are necessary for two to four weeks.

Acupuncture

Although this is not a classic, mainstream treatment, some of my patients claim great results. If you do seek this type of therapy, consider that you are not truly addressing the problems of inflammation and abnormal motion. If acupuncture does help the pain, then consider other therapies that address the problem in addition to acupuncture.

Shock Wave Therapy

Extracorporeal Shock Wave Therapy (ESWT) is a new therapy for plantar fasciitis. Strong sound waves penetrate the heel area and stimulate a healing response by the body. This is done as an outpatient procedure and is used only in resistant plantar fasciitis cases. There are some side effects and complications including bruising of the skin, swelling, pain, numbness or tingling, and even rupture of the plantar fascia, but they are rare.

Surgery

Surgery is the last resort. Less than 10% of patients will need to have heel surgery. Usually six to twelve months of conservative care is attempted before surgery is considered. There are two types of procedures.

One type is to make a small incision at the heel, cutting the fascia and removing the bone spur (if there is a spur). This type of surgery usually involves a walking cast, a cast boot or sometimes crutches for four to six weeks.

The other type of surgery is done endoscopically with small incisions. The fascia is visualized by looking in with a very small camera. Only the fascia is cut, and the bone spur is left alone. (Remember my discussion earlier about the bone spur not causing the pain). The results with this surgery are very good and the healing time may be reduced, but a cast boot or walking cast for four weeks is still necessary.

The Bottom Line

Try all the conservative therapy first. Make a good effort to perform the daily treatment. Don't wait too long before seeing your doctor and getting started. Know that this condition takes many months before it will be healed completely. Surgery is the last resort. Fortunately, few people will need surgery.

10

Diabetes

Overview

As you may know, *diabetes* is an increase in sugar (glucose) in the blood system. Some people develop this disease early in life and some develop it later in life. Diabetes can have a significant effect on your feet. The increase in blood sugar causes damage to the blood vessels and to the nerves.

Blood Vessels

The blood vessels in your body are the arteries (which carry blood from your heart to your feet) and the veins (which carry blood from your feet to your heart). When the feet are swollen, it means that the blood is not traveling from the feet up to the heart through the veins. When the muscles in the legs contract they help pump the blood back up to the heart. When you have cold feet, and no *pulses*, your blood is having problems getting from your heart to your feet.

Circulation is the blood traveling from the heart to the feet and back again

By far, the worst circulation problem occurs when the blood does not get from the heart to the feet. Bad circulation to your feet is usually a result of diabetes, smoking, poor health or poor eating habits. It could be due to all of the above. In diabetes, the high sugar levels contribute to hardened arteries that don't allow nutrients into the tissue. A diabetic's artery will clog up faster than a non-diabetic.

When blood can't get down to the feet, it can't deliver the vital nutrients the body needs. It can also cause cold feet and pain. With poor circulation to the feet, healing a simple cut on the foot is very difficult for the body. There is an increased chance of infection because the body can't deliver the nutrients it needs to fight the infection.

Nerves

The nerves in the body tell you what types of sensation you are feeling. They also tell your muscles when to move. Nerves can tell the difference between hot, cold, pain, light touch, position and vibration. There is a reason for pain. Pain tells you something is wrong. Pain experienced in the foot is sent as a message to the brain. This information is processed and then the brain sends a signal to the foot to adjust for that pain. For example, normally if you step on something sharp, you pull your foot off of the sharp object. If you don't have sensation in your foot and you step on something sharp, then you will not pull your foot away.

In diabetics, the nerves lose the ability to sense pain. There are many theories why this happens:
• The blood supply (as discussed above) is decreased and the nerves cannot function without an adequate blood supply.

• The increase in sugar in the body causes the nerves to

Those Aching Feet

malfunction.
- There are loses of the specific enzymes that are needed to enable nerve function.
- Diabetics have more free radicals in their system as a result of the increased sugar. This causes a malfunction of the nerves.

Regardless of the reason, the result is the same: loss of sensation to the feet. Approximately 60% of diabetics over 60 years old will develop a loss of sensation in their feet. Approximately 70% of diabetics with foot ulcers did not consider themselves "at risk" for foot ulcerations. Knowing more about your feet and how to take care of them is the key to prevention!

What You See and Feel

The problem is usually that most diabetics don't feel anything. With a loss of sensation, the most common sensation is numbness. This usually makes it difficult to remember the feet. Typically, this is called "stocking glove neuropathy" because it starts out at the toes and progresses up the legs evenly, as if you were putting on a stocking.

There can be a painful loss of sensation called painful diabetic *neuropathy*. Patients with this type of neuropathy have tingling, burning and sharp pains, usually at night or at rest. The pain is less when walking. They find it difficult to sleep at night, and the sheet covers can be quite uncomfortable.

Foot ulcers are another common diabetic problem. A foot ulcer is a break in the skin and appears like an open sore. This is a fairly difficult problem to notice when it is on the bottom of your foot. How many people do you know who can bring their foot up to eye level and examine the bottom? Most likely, not many. Most people will notice drainage on their socks or bed sheets or in their shoes as the first sign. Some will notice redness creeping to the top of the foot, if it gets infected. Sometimes the ulcer goes unnoticed until it

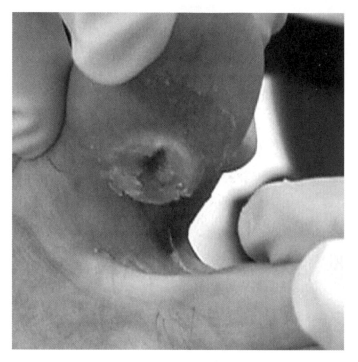

Figure 10-1 ulcer on bottom of the big toe

becomes infected. Once infected, redness will show on the top of the foot accompanied by drainage, pus and a foul odor.

How It's Diagnosed

Neuropathy (loss of sensation or nerve function) is diagnosed with a few simple tests by your doctor. She or he may test for vibration with a tuning fork or use a Q-Tip to test the difference between sharp and dull. An important test is the *protective threshold* test. This test is done with a small mono-filament wire. This wire is very thin and can barely be felt. This test lets the doctor know your risk of developing an ulcer. Basically, there is a *threshold* between feeling some sensation and feeling no sensation. Once an individual passes the threshold into "no sensation", then the nerves will no longer act protective. At this point, the nerves cannot protect the foot from developing an ulcer.

An ulcer is fairly easy to diagnose. Any break or hole in the skin is defined as an ulcer. The trick is to find out why one is having the ulcer. It may be due to a bone spur, too much pressure, abnormal motion, poor circulation or high blood pressure. Some ulcers have too much callous tissue, and the callous tissue needs to be removed to find the ulcer underneath.

What Else Could It Be?

There are many other conditions that can cause neuropathy. Diabetes is the most common, but other conditions include certain medications, frostbite, alcoholism and some sexually transmitted diseases. If you have tingling, numbness or burning in your feet that occurs mostly at night, and you are not a diabetic, see your physician.

Ulcers can be mistaken for callouses. This is quite common. Callous tissue can build up and cover an ulceration. The two are easily differentiated by shaving off the top layer of callous.

What You Can Do About It

The most important thing you can do is maintain a healthy lifestyle. Eat healthy, keep your blood sugar near a normal level, do not smoke, do get exercise and do decrease stress. All of these factors contribute to the overall health of your body and your feet.

Do not shave the top layer of a callous at home. Visit your doctor!

The second most important thing is prevention. Once you have an ulcer, it puts you at risk for developing an infection or possibly gangrene. Either of these can lead to amputation. The chances of developing ulcers and infections increases once you have neuropathy or poor circulation.

The best treatment for you is to prevent the problem before it starts. Here's how:

Check your feet everyday!

This is an absolute necessity. If you can't reach your feet, have a friend or family member check your feet for cuts, sores, bruises, openings or areas of irritation. Alternatively, put a mirror on the floor and put your foot over it. Make sure you check between your toes. Very moist areas, white areas or red areas are bad. Foot fungus will show up as patchy, scaly white areas between your toes or on the bottom of the feet. Check for irritated areas with redness or swelling. Also check for infection. Redness, pus and drainage are signs of infection. And while you are inspecting your feet, check your toes for ingrown nails.

Check your shoes before you put your feet in them.

Small pebbles or rocks can hide in the shoe. Put your hand in first and check it before you place your foot into the shoe.

Don't walk around barefoot or in sandals.

Splinters and needles can be hidden in the carpet and can puncture a foot without sensation. Punctures can go unnoticed. Unprotected feet can be more damaged when bumped or hit against furniture.

> The best treatment is to prevent the problem before it even starts.

Watch out for folds in your socks.

Believe it or not, small folds in the socks can lead to ulcers and infections. Rough seams in the socks can also cause areas of irritation that may lead to skin breakdown and ulceration.

Dry your feet and between toes after showers

Increased moisture between your toes can lead to the skin breaking down. This will eventually lead to an ulcer between the toes. Ulcers between the toes are very difficult to cure.

Don't be a victim of fashion

High fashion shoes usually lead to a high number of problems in the feet. When buying shoes, select footwear that is soft and flexible and allows for cush-

One day a diabetic with severe neuropathy came in for her routine appointment. She complained of a "sore" on her left foot. As I went to examine her left foot, a shiny silver piece of metal caught my eye. "Do you mean your right foot?" "No" she replied. "I'm concerned about the left" As she pointed. "This callous or sore is bothersome." I examined her right foot and pulled out a shiny, silver tack...I then said, "I am more concerned about your right foot." She had no idea that she had been walking around with a tack in her right foot.

ioning. Make sure they don't fold up into a ball. That is too flexible. But also be sure that the shoes are not too rigid. Confirm that your new shoes are wide enough. Don't buy shoes that are too wide or too long which can cause a lot of slipping and may lead to areas of irritation, skin breakdown and ulceration.

Ask your doctor about the possibility of your insurance company paying for extra-depth shoes with custom insoles. These shoes will take the pressure off your feet.

Is your bath water too hot?
Check the bath water with your hand before you put your foot in it. If you have neuropathy, the temperature your foot feels is much different from the temperature your hand feels. Make sure to check the temperature by inserting your hand into the water to wrist depth. This will be much more accurate then testing the water with your foot.

Don't use a heating pad on your feet.
Because of a diabetics reduced foot sensation, you may not even notice the heating pad causing burns on your feet.

Don't use any medication on the skin
Do not use medicated corn pads or any medicated pads from the local drug store. These medicated pads are usually not effective, and may cause a chemical burn on the surrounding skin. Don't use any medication on the skin unless you are instructed to by your physician.

Do not cut your own toenails
If you have loss of sensation or decreased blood supply, make sure to have a podiatrist trim your toenails.

Do not trim your own callous or corns
If you have a loss of sensation or low blood supply have your podiatrist trim your corns or callouses.

Stop smoking
This applies to everyone, especially diabetics.
- Smoking causes the blood vessels to shrink.
- Smoking contributes to clogging of the arteries.
- Smoking also makes it more difficult for the nutrients in the blood to get to the areas they are needed.
- Diabetes + Smoking = Disaster

If you don't have neuropathy or poor circulation but you do have diabetes, all the above mentioned instructions may not apply to you. Still, you should definitely follow all the guidelines and be aware of the potential problems. I recommend consulting your podiatrist for advice. Be sure to make a yearly visit for a foot examination. If you have neuropathy or poor circulation, you should see a podiatrist every two months.

STOP SMOKING!

What You Can Do About It: Neuropathy

There are many treatments for painful neuropathy. Unfortunately, not all of them are effective. Some people respond to some treatments better than others. The following is a partial list of common treatments.

Capsacian (Zostrix®) cream
Some patients have a significant amount of relief; some find that capsacian increases the pain. This cream is now available at the drug store at strengths up to .075%. Be careful using this cream, wear gloves and do not get this in your eyes. Carefully wash your hands afterwards. To apply, place a small amount on your feet at night, and then cover with a sock. Some people will

experience a small burning sensation.

An alternative to Capsacian cream, is an inexpensive home remedy consisting of two teaspoons of powdered chili pepper and some baby powder placed in a sock. Shake the sock and then wear it at night. You can also mix chili-powder and body lotion.

Anti-inflammatory medications or Tylenol®
Most patients do not have complete relief when using these medications, but many patients notice some pain relief.

Elavil® (amitriptyline)
It has been shown to help relieve nerve pain at lower doses. This is still used as an anti-depressant medication at higher doses. Many people have a significant amount of relief by taking Elavil® before they go to sleep. Available by prescription only.

Topical gels
There are a few pharmacies that will mix topical medications to treat painful neuropathy. The formula usually consists of some combination of amitriptyline, baclofen® and ketamine and sometimes ketoprofen.

Neurontin® Controversy?

A controversy surrounding Neurontin® developed a few years ago. A whistle-blower from the company that provides Neurontin® stated that the company promoted the drug for "off-label" uses not approved by the FDA and downplayed the side effects, such as very low blood pressure. This is something to be concerned about and to discuss with your physician.

I have found that many patients tolerate Neurontin® quite well at lower doses. An article in *Clinical Theraputics*, January 2003, reviewed five randomized, placebo-controlled trials (the gold standard of studies in the medical field). They concluded that gabapentin (Neurontin®) was an effective treatment in painful neuropathy, with very few mild side effects. The bottom line is that you need to consult your doctor, be aware of any side effects you are experiencing and start with low doses if you consider taking this medication.

Many patients find relief of the burning pain with use of this gel combination. It is by prescription only.

Neurontin® (gabapentin)

This medication is FDA approved only for seizures. It was later found that (in much smaller doses) it also helps with nerve pain. It's available by prescription only.

Gamma linolenic acid (GLA)

GLA is an essential fatty acid, a substance that is essential to the body that cannot be made by the body. It has been shown to indirectly affect the blood vessels, the clotting ability of the body and the body's healing system. Diabetics often have low levels of natural Gamma linolenic acid. GLA has also been shown to help reverse some of the effects of neuropathy. The jury is still out on GLA. There have been many studies that show it's positive effects, but GLA is not yet a mainstream form of therapy. There are very few side effects associated with GLA, but it is always a good idea to check with your physician before you proceed with taking any supplements.

An effective dose of GLA is 360-480mg per day. Starting with the dosage recommended on the bottle is the best way to start with the medication. Slowly increase your dose over the next week until you reach 480mg. This will allow your body to adjust, and see if you have any side effects. Doses up to 2,800mg appear to be well tolerated. The trick is finding a capsule that contains the higher dose amount of GLA. Make sure you read the back of each container to find the correct amounts. You can also find GLA as currant seed oil, primrose oil or borage oil.

Alpha-lipoic acid (ALA)

This is another supplement that has been shown to have some positive effects on neuropathy. Alpha-lipoic acid is a free radical scavenger, and considered an antioxidant. Most have heard the term "free radical

Note

If all therapies have failed then your primary care doctor may send you to see a neurologist.

Those Aching Feet

When the body *oxidizes*, it creates oxygen molecules that are not bonded to anything. For instance: oxygen and two hydrogen bond together to make water (H_2O). When oxygen has an extra charge and is not bonded to anything else it is called a free-radical. It is free to attach to anything. When these free-radicals roam the body, they can attach to areas they shouldn't. This usually results in abnormal events. Free-radical scavengers are molecules that can attract free-radicals, attach to them and then flush them out of the system. The term anti-oxidant is most likely familiar to you. This term describes the free-radical scavengers. Alpha-lipoic acid is an anti-oxidant and a free-radical scavenger. Diabetics have increased oxidative stress, meaning more of the oxygen radicals are being formed and are floating around the body, causing problems. One possible problem can be with the blood flow. Another possible problem is with the nerve function.

scavenger", but few people know what it means. (explained above) Alpha-lipoic acid has been shown to help deter the free-radicals, and decrease the problems with nerve function. The recommended dose is 800mg a day. You need to be warned that neither ALA nor GLA are mainstream therapies for treatment of diabetic neuropathy. Some studies have shown only modest improvement and have noted that these supplements can be quite expensive.

What You Can Do About It: Ulcers

There are many treatments for ulcers. The treatments typically aim at the type of ulceration. There are hundreds of wound gels for diabetic ulcers, but many of them are the same. Ulcers are not a medical problem that you can take care of by yourself. See your physician.

Some ulcers need *debridement* (taking off the top layer of dead skin) and others do not. Ulcers that drain and ooze require dressings that can pull fluid out like "wet to dry" dressings or absorbing foam-type dressings. Dry ulcers require moisture with creams. Ulcers that are not pink may require an "enzymatic debriding ointment". This means that the ointment will help take away the bad tissue and help to replace it with new tissue. New and expensive medications can help grow new cells. If an ulcer has been there for many months or years, than x-rays need to be taken to make sure there is no underlying bone infection. A bone scan may be needed. If you smoke, your ulcer will not heal. If your sugars are high, your ulcer will not heal. If there is an underlying infection, your ulcer will not heal. If you are walking and putting all your pressure on it, most likely that ulcer will not heal. There are many things to consider when treating an ulcer. Please see your physician as soon as possible if you develop an ulcer.

If you are diabetic and have either neuropathy or poor circulation, than you should be eligible for diabetic shoes and custom inserts. MediCare will pay for this service for you every year. Many insurance companies will do the same. Ask your physician.

The Bottom Line

If you are a diabetic and have either poor circulation or neuropathy, you need to see your podiatrists once every two months for routine care. You need to check your feet everyday. You need to lead a healthy lifestyle, maintaining your blood sugar level and exercising daily. You must stop smoking. Preventing diabetic foot problems is easier than treating them.

Flat Feet

pes pla·no val·gus

Overview

Flatfeet also known as "low arch feet" are medically referred to as *pes plano valgus*. They are fairly common among the general population. Just because an individual has flatfeet does not necessarily mean that the individual will have foot problems. There are many different types of feet. Some feet have extremely high arches and others have extremely low arches. The rest of the population has feet that fit somewhere in between. Individuals who have extremely low arches are the ones that will have multiple foot problems as a result of the low arch. These types of flat feet are medically termed *pathologic pes plano valgus*. Individuals with low arches, which are not extreme, usually have mild foot problems. Some individuals with flatfeet never have foot problems. Many great athletes have flatfeet. Most people with flatfeet were born with that foot type, but some develop flatfeet as a result of arthritis, injury or disease.

What You See and Feel

The arch is low and sometimes it may touch the floor. The heels are turned out and the ankles turned in when seen from the back. Many times the Achilles tendon makes a C-shape curvature, being convex on the inside. Extra creases may form on the outside of the foot below the ankle. Many times the feet turn out (duck-walking).

Some of the problems associated with flatfeet are *plantar fasciitis, Achilles tendonitis, bunions, hammertoes, corns, callouses* and *posterior tibialis tendonitis*. Many of these conditions are discussed in other chapters. Arch pain is a common complaint and usually a result of *fasciitis* or *posterior tibialis tendonitis*. Tendonitis is common on almost any area of the foot, but the most common at the Achilles tendon. Usually the pain is the most severe when the foot hits the ground in the morning, and it is generally localized to the back of the heel and at the Achilles tendon. Sometimes a small mass is felt at that area. Posterior tibialis tendonitis is at the inside of the arch and sometimes can be the cause of the low arch in extreme cases. There is usually a bone that is prominent and 'sticks out'. This is where most of the pain occurs.

Patients may experience back pain because of their foot position. This is usually in the case of extreme flatfeet. When the foot collapses too much, it cause the knee to rotate in and hence the hip. This causes abnormal walking and can affect the back. Leg pain, achiness and fatigue can be a result of flatfeet. Some individuals also develop knee pain or hip pain.

Infants will always have flatfeet. The arch develops between ages 4 to 8 years of age. Severe flatfeet will be noticeable before this age and may affect walking. Infants normally start walking at 8-14 months of age. When the feet are very flat, or the child is tripping and falling, or the infant hasn't begun walking after 14 months visit your physician. Flatfeet may be causing these problems.

How It's Diagnosed

Most individuals will come in with a complaint of flatfeet and sore arches. Many people may have flatfeet, but only some will have problems related to the flatfeet. To diagnose a pathologic pes plano valgus foot, the physician must examine the foot standing and not standing, as well as observe the gait (walking). While standing, the most important anatomy to assess is the heel position. The physician will note whether it is everted or inverted. When walking, the physician can assess how much abnormal pronation a patient has in their feet. Pronation is the rolling in of the foot during walking. A certain amount of pronation is necessary, an abnormal amount can cause problems.

What Else Could It Be?

Since there are many problems associated with flatfeet, it is important to find out what the problem is, and what is causing it. Correcting the flatfoot may be the treatment for many of the conditions listed above. Sometimes arthritis may be causing the flatfoot. If the foot collapses suddenly, it could be a result of the tendon rupturing or possibly a charcot foot. A *charcot foot* usually occurs in the diabetic (but can occur in anyone who has a loss of sensation) and involves collapsing of the joints due to multiple tiny fractures in the bones. This is not uncommon in the diabetic with a loss of sensation.

What You Can Do About It

Many of the treatments have already been described in other chapters for the problems associated with flatfeet. Here are a few methods that may help prevent flatfeet problems. First, buy a correct pair of shoes. Most people wear their shoes too tight and too small. Many shoes available are not wide enough for the average foot. Americans, in general, wear their shoes one size too small. Listed below are the seven tests that you should use when buying shoes. I never recommend a specific type of shoe because shoes are so individual; what is right for one person, may not be right for the next person. Shoe companies put out many different styles of shoes every year. One year a company may have a great shoe, and the next year, it may be a poor shoe. Spending a lot of money does not guarantee a good shoe.

Evaluating New Shoes

Shoe bends only where the foot bends
- See figures 11-1 and 11-2
- You don't want the shoe to fold up into a ball.
- You don't want the shoe to bend in the arch.
- You don't want the shoe to not bend at all.

High and moderately stiff heel counter
- The heel counter is the back of the shoe that surrounds the heel.
- The heel counter helps to stabilize the heel and protect it.
- The heel counter should not be too rigid or it will be uncomfortable and cause blistering.
- It should also not be too flexible, or it won't allow for support.
- Test the heel counter by squeezing it and pushing it forward.

Large enough toe box
- The toe box is the front of the shoe where the toes sit.
- Make sure that it is not only wide enough, but also high enough to allow room for the toes.
- Most fashionable shoes have been too narrow in the toe box. Luckily, wider toe boxes are available now.

Wedged heel
- Make sure that the heel is raised slightly higher than the front of the shoe.
- This is not a "high heel" shoe, but has a slightly higher heel in the back than in the front, making a

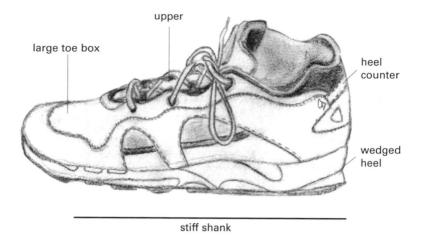

large toe box

upper

heel counter

wedged heel

stiff shank

Figure 11-1 shoe characteristics

wedge shape.
- This helps to take pressure off of the Achilles tendon and the arch.
- With athletic shoes, make sure you place your hand in the heel to see how high the heel is. Many of the styles will exaggerate the lift with their design

Stiff upper
- The upper is the top part of the shoe that connects with the toe box and the laced section.
- If you can put your hand in the shoe in the front and shift from side to side without displacing the material much, then it is a stiff upper.
- If you can put your hand in the shoe and push the material freely from one side to the other, then it is too flexible.
- This is important because the flexible material will allow your foot to actually slide off of the insole while you're walking.

Arch support
- For the flat-footed person, having an arch support can cause more pain. It feels like a ball under the arch.

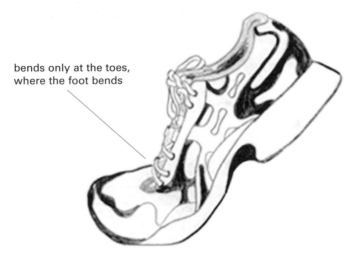

bends only at the toes,
where the foot bends

Figure 11-2 shoe characteristics

- A small arch support is necessary and helpful for most people.
- Removable insoles with a small arch support built-in are the best

Fit and comfort
- This is by far the most important aspect of proper shoe selection.
- Each person is individual and each foot is individual.
- If you find a brand and a shoe you like, write it down and stick with it.
- Walk around the shoe store in both shoes.
- Take the shoes home and wear them inside for a few days to make sure they fit well.
- Look for areas of irritation on your feet.

What You Can Do About It: Orthotics

Many people with flatfeet can benefit from *orthotics*. Orthotics are devices that are custom molded to your feet with foam or plaster. The mold of your foot is then used to develop a device that is custom to your feet and helps to correct any abnormal motion. In most cases, an orthotic is hard and made to control motion. It

10 Points of Proper Shoe Fit

A list of recommendations on proper shoe fit was produced jointly by the American Orthopedic Foot and Ankle Society, the Pedorthic Footwear Association and the National Shoe Retailers Association in a pamphlet titled 10 Points of Proper Shoe Fit. They are as follows:

1. Sizes vary among shoe brands and styles. Do not select shoes by the size marked inside the shoe; judge the shoe by how it fits on your foot.

2. Select a shoe that conforms as nearly as possible to the shape of your foot.

3. Have your feet measured regularly. The size of your feet changes as you grow older.

4. Have BOTH feet measured. Most people have one foot larger than the other. Fit to the largest foot.

5. Fit at the end of the day, when your feet are the largest.

6. Stand during the fitting process and check that there is adequate space (3/8 to 1/2 inch) for your longest toe at the end of each shoe.

7. Make sure the ball of your foot fits snugly into the widest part (ball pocket) of the shoe.

8. Do not purchase shoes that feel too tight, expecting them to "stretch" to fit.

9. Your heel should fit comfortably in the shoe with a minimum amount of slippage.

10. Walk in the shoe to make sure it fits and feels right (fashionable shoes CAN be comfortable!).

Shoes have been a growing culprit in the development of deformities of the foot, especially the front of the foot. Getting the proper fit is important.

is not soft like an arch support, but there may be a soft cover. When I take an impression casting of someone's foot, I hold the foot in it's neutral position. This is the position the foot should be in. It is lined up under the knee, and the central line of gravity should travel down the leg through the center of the foot. When standing, the flatfoot collapses and does not hold the neutral position. The center of gravity is shifted and travels down to the inside of the foot. The knee rotates inward, and places a rotation force on the hip and back. Most of the abnormal motion in the foot comes from the back of the foot. Attempts to hold up an arch, at the arch, are unsuccessful in flatfeet because the arch collapse starts back at the heel area. When the foot is in a neutral position, it is also more stable. As it turns in, or pronates, it becomes unstable and 'floppy', spreading out and becoming wide. All of these factors can be controlled with orthotics.

As an aside, I would like to mention that there are different types of orthotics. There are *accommodative orthotics* and *functional orthotics*. Accommodative orthotics are usually made by stepping into a foam box or plaster mold. This type of orthotic accommodates the foot. It is soft and flexible. It is not made to control motion. Functional orthotics are rigid and don't bend. Sometimes they are made by stepping into a mold, but most times they are made by casting the foot in the neutral position, which requires the patient to be sitting or lying down. Functional orthotics are the best orthotic for flatfeet, and the cast should be taken in the neutral position. Throughout this chapter I have been referring to functional orthotics.

In extreme cases when the foot is resistant to conservative therapy and the flatfoot is severe, surgery can be done. This is only recommended when the pain is severe and limiting walking and daily activities. Most of the surgeries developed to treat flatfoot are complicated and involve a foot reconstruction. Many times bones are broken and re-set, tendons are transposed from one part of the foot to the other, the Achilles tendon may be lengthened and some joints can be fused. Undergoing this type of surgery results in about two to three months off of your feet, and a six month recovery period. Expect a year before functioning at an optimal level again. The results are quite good for these surgeries if they are done properly.

The Bottom Line

If you are having pain at the arch and feel as if you have flatfeet, first try to find a good pair of shoes. If you don't get relief from the shoes, ask your physician about orthotics. Make sure you see a specialist trained in foot biomechanics. All podiatrists and most foot and ankle orthopedic specialists will have this training, but is not common for orthopedists to fit patients with orthotics. Most chiropractors will also have this training; and some may be able to fit you with a functional orthotic. *Pedorthists* do not have training in biomechanics, but have extensive knowledge about shoes and inserts. They can usually mold an excellent accommodative orthotic. If you have flatfeet, make sure that the person taking your foot impression is placing plaster around your feet, and not using a step-in mold. If a step-in mold is used, the foot is held in position. A step-in foam mold, used for accommodative orthotics, will take a cast of your foot in the incorrect position. This type of orthotic is great for accommodation which is especially useful for diabetics. As with other foot problems, surgery is the last choice, and only necessary in extreme cases.

12

Cysts

gan·gli·o·nic cysts

Overview

A *ganglionic cyst* is a fluid filled sac that usually comes from either the lining of a tendon or a joint. There can be many causes for ganglion cysts, but the most common cause is excess stress in one area, usually from a shoe rubbing on the top of the foot. This can weaken the lining of the tendon or joint capsule and cause an outpouching of fluid. Any repetitive irritation can cause this. Some *ganglions* will be formed for no reason at all, and others have an associated bone spur beneath them. Certain foot types may have an abnormal shape that causes excess shoe irritation and can lead to a ganglionic cyst.

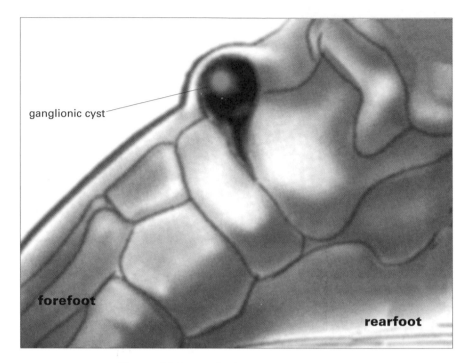

ganglionic cyst

forefoot

rearfoot

Figure 12-1 ganglionic cyst

What You See and Feel

Usually there is a small lump on the top of the foot. This lump is usually soft, but can be firm in some instances. If you push on the lump it might be tender, but usually painful when constantly irritated by a shoe. It is usually freely moveable. It may be above a nerve and result in a burning sensation, tingling or numbness. With an increase in dependency of the feet, there is usually an increase in size of the ganglion. Weather can also cause changes in the size.

How It's Diagnosed

A ganglionic cyst is diagnosed by a good history and physical exam by your physician. X-rays might be taken (if the cyst occurs in a certain area of the foot) to rule out a bone spur. Fluid may be taken out of the cyst and sent to the laboratory for examination if the cyst appears abnormal. Usually a clear jelly-like fluid con-

Those Aching Feet

firms the diagnosis of a cyst and a laboratory evaluation is not needed.

What Else Could It Be?

There are a few different types of lumps that can form on the foot. In most cases a ganglionic cyst is fairly easy to identify. A *synovial cyst* is a type of ganglionic cyst which mainly appears over joint areas. Sometimes there may be fluid leaking from this cyst. *Nodules* that occur over joints may also appear like a ganglion. A *fibrotic* (scar tissue) mass may also look like a ganglion but it will be firmer and attached to deeper tissue. A *sebacious* cyst is a mass that is filled with an oily fluid or with dead tissue. Rarely, a sarcoma (cancer) can develop on the foot and appear like a cyst. If a cyst increases in size or pain quickly, be sure to see your physician immediately.

What You Can Do About It?

Do not take a bible and smash the cyst. It's an incorrect age old treatment for these cysts, as well as the origin of the term "bible bump", that can potentially lead to further problems. I know it sounds unbelievable, but I have actually had patients attempt to find a cyst remedy using the bible.

Do not use the "bible bump" technique, it could lead to further problems.

Placing padding around the cyst may help with the pressure. Find appropriate shoes that allow space for the cyst. Your physician can remove the fluid in the cyst and may inject steroids into the area, but many times these treatments are unsuccessful.

The next step is surgery. I only recommend it for those with pain and limited walking caused by the cyst. Surgery will usually remove the cyst, but there is a small chance of recurrence. The surgery involves removing the cyst (and bone spur if there is one) and then remaining in a surgical shoe for two to three weeks. You can walk immediately after the surgery, and the pain is typically not severe. Within three to four weeks you will be back in regular shoes, participating in your regular activity.

The Bottom Line

Try padding and switching shoes first. Lacing the shoes loosely in the area may decrease the irritation. If you have no relief, removing the fluid and a steroid injection is the next step. This often fails and surgery is needed, but only if the cyst **increases your pain and limits your activity**.

Neuroma

Overview

A *neuroma* is an inflamed nerve. It can occur at any
point along a nerve, but typically occurs in areas of
stress or irritation. In the foot, the most common place
for a neuroma is between the third and fourth
metatarsals in the forefoot. Most people complain of
pain on the bottom of the foot that shoots out to the
third and fourth toe. Neuromas can also occur between
the second and third toe, as well as on a bunion. The
most common neuroma is called a Morton's neuroma.
This neuroma occurs between the third and fourth toe.
There are many theories for the development of neuromas in this area. First, this area is the place where two
nerves merge, forming a slightly larger nerve. It is postulated that this large nerve has a higher chance of
being irritated. There are two columns to the foot which

can sometimes act independently. The third and fourth metatarsals separate these two columns. Some say this contributes to increased irritation. In some individuals, the two metatarsals are closer together and this aggravates the nerve. Others feel that there is a ligament between the metatarsals that places pressure on the nerve and causes irritation. Although there appears to be many theories for the cause of a neuroma, there is a general agreement that a certain foot type causes an abnormal motion in the foot that leads to irritation of the nerve. Generally, the pain will appear after increased time spent on the feet, but can also appear after an injury.

What You See and Feel

The pain is usually sharp and localized to the ball of the foot. Pain may shoot out to the toes, particularly the third and fourth toe. It may feel as if you are walking on a marble or a cord. Stopping, sitting down and rubbing or massaging the foot may help the pain. The foot can remain painful and achy even if there is no pressure on the foot.

How It's Diagnosed

The neuroma is diagnosed purely by good questioning and a physical exam of the foot by your physician. Pressing on certain areas of the foot will reproduce the pain. A certain test will actually cause a clicking sound that pops the nerve out from between the bones. The clicking sound associated with pain shooting to the toes is diagnostic for a Morton's neuroma. An x-ray can be helpful in ruling out other conditions. In some cases the neuroma can be confused with inflammation of the joints at the forefoot. Commonly, both of the conditions exist at the same time. It may be necessary to inject local anesthetic into the area in order to figure out the diagnosis. Other tests are usually not necessary.

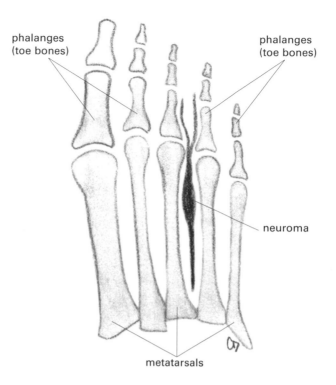

phalanges
(toe bones)

phalanges
(toe bones)

neuroma

metatarsals

Figure 13-1 morton's neuroma

What Else Could It Be?

The most common misdiagnosis is *capsulitis*. Capsulitis is the inflammation of the joint capsule and it can commonly occur in the forefoot. The pain may be quite similar to the neuroma pain. Many times these conditions occur together because the foot becomes over-stressed and many structures in the area become irritated. An injection with numbing medication in the area may be necessary to help distinguish between the two problems. A *bursa* in the same area may cause similar types of pain.

What You Can Do About It

The first step in treatment is to decrease your activity and impact on the foot. To start the healing, the irritation of the nerve must be decreased. In association with

13: Neuroma

decreasing impact activity on the foot, neuroma pads can be placed under the forefoot. These pads will help decrease irritation to the nerve. Ice will also help to decrease inflammation and so will anti-inflammatory medications. For certain foot types, orthotics may be necessary. A steroid injection will help to decrease the inflammation in the area. No more than four injections should be given in the same area in a 12 months period. If two injections have not helped it is not likely that a third injection will make any difference. More aggressive therapy includes soft casts and the use of crutches.

If the conservative therapy has not helped, surgery is the next option. Surgery involves removing the nerve. It is a fairly simple and short procedure. The recovery involves wearing a surgical shoe for two weeks afterwards. Crutches are not necessary after surgery in most cases. Full recovery takes four to six weeks. Numbness between the toes after surgery is unavoidable. One of the more common complications of the surgery is the development of a stump neuroma. The nerve can become irritated at the site where it was cut and cause pain. I only recommend the surgery after all of the conservative therapy has been tried.

The Bottom Line

Visit your physician and try the conservative therapy. If you receive no relief from the therapy you may need a steroid injection. Continue the conservative therapy after the injection. If the pain is still continuing, then consider surgery.

14

Athletes

Introduction

The very reason I went into podiatric medicine was because I was so interested in sports medicine. I was interested in how the lower extremity functioned and I was fascinated by the biomechanics of the feet and legs. Part of my interest is due to the fact that I have had many foot and leg problems over the years, including being pigeon-toed, wearing orthotics for years, and having chronic ankle sprains, ankle fractures, heel pain, arch pain and shin splints.

I'm a doctor and also an athlete. I often feel that the medical approach for an athlete should be slightly varied from the approach for non-athletes. I have competed in sprint distance triathlons, 10Ks, half and full marathons, century cycling rides, mountain bike

An athlete includes both amateurs and professionals. It's people involved in both individual or team activities. He or she may be involved competitively or recreationally. They may be part of a league, club, team or they just do it on their own. The events can be sports, endurance races, games or just fun. Events range from badminton to basketball, jump-roping to jogging, martial arts to motocross, rowing to rugby. Some events are very physically demanding, some require great strength or speed, while others require more precision and hand eye coordination. An athlete is anyone who participates in physical events or sports.

races and ski races as well as played soccer, tennis, racquetball, swimming and softball. I am no stranger to injury. I've had casts on my legs and been on crutches more than once. I particularly know how frustrating an injury can be for an athlete. There is the aggravation of interrupted training and the frustration of being sedentary. There is a urge to get back to the activity before you are ready....Believe me, I know, I have been there myself many times. I understand this frustration and incorporate it when I am talking to my patients who are athletes and regular exercisers. I know how difficult it is to break a routine, to stop the activity, to just slow down, to rest.

This chapter is going to highlight a few foot conditions common in athletes and some tips to help you avoid returning to your activity too soon, thereby bypassing unnecessary complications and problems.

ACHILLES TENDONITIS
Overview

Tendonitis is the inflammation of a tendon, usually at or close to it's *insertion*. There are two types of Achilles tendonitis. There is *insertional Achilles tendonitis* and the standard *Achilles tendonitis*. Insertional tendonitis occurs at the insertion of the Achilles tendon into the heel bone. The standard Achilles tendonitis occurs about two to three inches above the insertion. Both of these conditions usually develop as a result of overuse or over stressing the area. Typically, starting a new activity or changing an activity will stress the area. Walking up and down hills puts the greatest amount of stress on the Achilles tendon. Any activity that doesn't allow the heel to touch the ground, puts excess stress on the tendon. Many people were either born with tight Achilles tendons or developed tight tendons. These individuals will have a natural predisposition for this condition.

Runners, incorporating hills into their regimen, can

develop Achilles tendonitis. Weight lifters overdoing calf exercises or performing squats incorrectly can develop this. Hiking, especially on hills with uneven terrain, can start this condition. Walkers adding distance, speed or hills to their routine can develop it. These are the most common factors that lead to tendonitis, but any new sport, change in a sport or overuse/overstress of a tendon can cause tendonitis. Even cycling, especially long distances, can lead to Achilles tendonitis. This can develop as a result of a dropped heel with steep hill climbing. Most of the injuries to the Achilles tendon are due to overuse. About 10% of pain in athletes, in the lower extremity, is due to Achilles tendon pain.

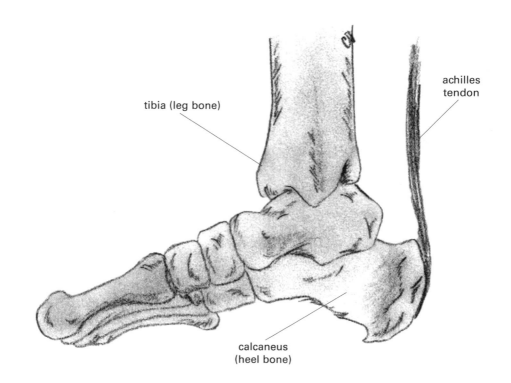

tibia (leg bone)

achilles tendon

calcaneus (heel bone)

Figure 14-1 diagram of the achilles tendon

ACHILLES TENDONITIS
What You See and Feel

For insertional tendonitis the pain is at the back of the heel bone. For standard Achilles tendonitis the pain is about two to three inches above the heel bone, at the tendon. Many times there is a small lump at the tendon which is tender to the touch. The area can appear swollen. The pain is usually felt in the morning, when first stepping out of bed. Then, it will work itself out, and gradually become more and more painful throughout the day. Sometimes, the pain only occurs at the beginning of the exercise. For instance, the first mile of a run will be painful, but then the pain seems to fade. The pain then returns, usually with a vengeance, at mile six or seven, and after the run.

ACHILLES TENDONITIS
How It's Diagnosed

The diagnosis is made by patient history and exam. There are no reliable or necessary tests that lead to the diagnosis. If a mass at the tendon is unusually large then, in rare cases, an MRI might be necessary.

ACHILLES TENDONITIS
What Else Could It Be?

There are a few conditions that have pain in the back of the heel.

Pump bump

Also called *Haglund's deformity*, this condition usually occurs between the age of 18-24 years of age and is most commonly seen in women. It is due to a combination of the foot shape and the shoe wear. Most people will notice a bump on the back of the heel bone which can become red and inflamed and painful with any pressure. Treatment is usually padding and switching shoes. In the case of those with extremely high arches, who are prone to this condition, surgery can be done, to remove the bump. Surgery is only done when pain is severe and has not responded to conservative therapy.

Achilles heel spur

Referred to as a *retrocalcaneal heel spur*, can occur at any age, but generally occurs at the ages of 35-65. When the Achilles tendon is over-stressed, the pull can cause a bone spur formation at the back of the heel. The tissues surrounding the spur can become inflamed, and any pressure can aggravate it. Usually the conservative therapies listed for Achilles tendonitis can treat this effectively, in association with padding around the spur. In the case of persistent pain, the bone spur can be removed in surgery. This may involve removing the Achilles tendon and reattaching it.

Bursa

A bursa is a small sac of fluid that develops because of abnormal pressure. At the back of the heel this condition is called *retrocalcaneal bursitis*. Sometimes, a *bursa* will develop in this area and cause pain. The bursa will commonly be associated with a heel spur. The treatments for this are the same as the treatments for Achilles tendonitis.

Pinched nerve

Also called *nerve entrapment*, this condition can be extremely painful, but is relatively rare. Nerve branches can be caught in scar tissue from an old surgery or injury to the area and become irritated. It is uncommon at the area of the Achilles tendon, but can be seen toward the inside heel area. The treatment may involve some of the listed therapies or may involve steroid injections.

Growth plate problems

Calcaneal apophysitis is a condition that commonly occurs in active children ages 8-14 years of age. The Achilles tendon attaches to the *apophysis* which is part of the heel bone in children. This bone does not *fuse* (become firmly attached to) the rest of the heel bone until 14-18 years of age. This is the heel bone's growth plate and it allows for growth of the bone. Since the tendon attaches to the smaller bone it can cause some movement at the growth plate. This is usually painful while playing sports, and happens more often in boys than in girls. The treatment is resting for two weeks (no sports) taking children's Motrin® on a daily basis, icing the area daily and placing a heel lift in the shoe. If the heel pain is resistant to therapy then the treatment may lead to casting or cast boots.

ACHILLES TENDONITIS
What You Can Do About It

The hardest part of all athletic injuries is the healing process . The healing that the foot needs to do will occur faster if there is no weight placed upon it. "Impossible" you say? Yes... But, this leads to the next step, which is to decrease activity. As I mentioned in the chapter on *plantar fasciitis* (Chapter 9), taking the recovery period in two week increments is the best way to approach the treatment. I also believe that the treatment is very individual. Some people may only need to taper their activity, while others should stop their activity completely. Below I discuss some guidelines for effectively dealing with tendonitis.

Stop the activity completely for five days. I usually recommend a full two weeks, but sometimes just five days will help considerably without compromising your activity level too much. Swim for exercise. Bike at low resistance at the gym and avoid the recumbent bike. If you bike outdoors, use the lowest gears when going up hills. Of course it is better to avoid hills if possible. Consider weight lifting, but avoid standing while lifting weights. It's important to avoid squats, calf lifts and quad bench presses.

Gradually return to your activities and usual activity level.

There are many areas that we tend to avoid when we focus on specific training, especially the upper body. Try to readjust your focus for a few weeks. Yoga is great for strengthening, give it a shot. Do avoid the downward dog and most lunges which can potentially overstretch the Achilles.

During your five days off, do the following conservative therapy. Ice twice a day at the back of the heel, for 20 minutes. Take anti-inflammatory medications. 800mg of ibuprofen three times a day is necessary to decrease pain and inflammation. Do not take this if you have stomach problems or any stomach irritation. (It is a good idea to consult a physician with such a high dose. Bleeding stomach ulcers have resulted from anti-inflammatory medications). Do calf stretches with your heel stretched out and front leg bent. Keep both heels on the floor. Do not hang your heel off of a step, this can further your injury. Only stretch until you feel a slight pain, and then back off. Hold for 1 minute and repeat three times. Add a heel lift to your regular shoe to take the pressure off of the Achilles tendon. Stretch your calf with a belt before you get out of bed in the morning, as described in the Chapter 9 (plantar fasciitis). Do not use heat on the area during these five days.

If you are feeling better after five days then gradually return to your activity. Do not return to 100% of your activity level too quickly. Start slowly. If you are a runner, try jogging a slow mile and assess how you feel. I know it does not sound like much of a workout, but you'll take about 1000 steps during that jog. Amazingly, that's all it takes to stress a weak, injured tendon. Make sure you wait 12 to 24 hours after exercising to assess the pain. Sometimes there is a delayed effect.

> Mid-distance and long-distance runners will create a force at the heel that is equal to as much as 200% of their body weight.

Cycling is a great cross-training exercise, but make sure to use a low resistance setting and pedal at higher RPMs. Do not drop the heel, to avoid adding additional force. Be sure you wear a heel lift in your biking shoe. If you do not have pain, then run a few miles the following day and then reassess. Keep using this method to test it out for a week, adding either mileage or intensity. At this point you should not add hills.

If you have pain at any time during the return, taper your routine accordingly. If you have a small amount of pain, then don't increase the mileage or intensity. Alternatively, give it a day's break while icing and taking anti-inflammatory medication. If you have a lot of pain when you return, then you should take off two full weeks from the activity. Talk to your physician to consider more aggressive therapy.

Some discomfort will be normal. Sharp pain is abnormal. After five days you can start what is called a friction rub. This involves rubbing across the tendon, at the painful or enlarged site for 20 minutes daily. (Do not rub down from the calf to the heel. After five days of reduced activity, contrast soaks will help (as described in Chapter 9).

If you successfully make it through the five days of rest, then the one week of gradual return without pain, it's time to start adding more intensity. Add hills if you wish at two weeks. Remember that tendonitis takes about six weeks to fully heal. You will be running, walking, or hiking on an injured tendon that has only partially healed at this point.

If the pain continues, you will need to take off another two week period starting with completely resting the foot again. If the pain still continues after the additional two weeks, make sure you see your physician. You might be developing a chronic injury that could take months to heal. If you haven't improved, ask your physician for other therapies. You may benefit from orthotics, as discussed in Chapter 11. A soft cast and crutches may be the added extra you need to decrease the inflammation and allow healing while forcing you to rest. A therapy that I do not recommend is a steroid injection in the area that has tendonitis. Steroid injections at the tendon can lead to tendon weakening, or rupture. If you do have a steroid injection, a cast or cast boot will be necessary for two weeks. Steroid injections near the heel bone are safer than higher on the tendon. Physical therapy with a "tens unit", ultrasound and contrast therapy can be a benefit as well. Surgery is usually not an option except for specific cases of tendonitis.

ACHILLES TENDONITIS
The Bottom Line

Act fast! If you let a condition like Achilles tendonitis continue on and on without rest or treatment, it will be extremely difficult to resolve. If you act fast and take the necessary time off, cross train, and then gradually return to your activity, your chances of healing quickly are much greater. Don't do the therapies half-way, this will just be a waste of your time. All or none to get the job done.

OTHER TYPES OF TENDONITIS

There are many areas of the foot that can develop tendonitis. Achilles tendonitis is by far the most common. *Peroneal tendonitis* is the inflammation of the tendon on the outside (lateral) of your foot. The tendonitis can be a result of any new increase in activity just like the development of Achilles tendonitis. Sometimes, there is a small bone in the same area that didn't fuse to the larger bone during development. This bone may cause irritation.

Posterior tibial tendonitis is the inflammation of the tendon at the inside of the arch. This can either be a result of the arch falling and placing stress on the tendon, or it can naturally stress and cause the arch to fall. This condition is outlined more in Chapter 9 on flatfeet. For athletes, the common posterior tibial tendonitis pain occurs right at the insertion of the tendon into the foot. This bone is called the *navicular* and it is a bone at the inside of the midfoot. (see figure 1-1) It usually is prominent (sticks out on the inside-*medially*) and also can be very tender and aggravated with any type of activity. Many people with this type of tendonitis have flatfeet. Along with the treatment listed for Achilles tendonitis, an orthotic is usually necessary.

PLANTAR FASCIITIS

I am going to refer you to Chapter 9 for most of the information on plantar fasciitis. Plantar fasciitis is quite common for runners, and when people start new sports like soccer or basketball. The pain that the athlete has can be different from that described in Chapter 9. Patients with fasciitis commonly have pain at the first step in the morning. However, athletes generally tend to have the pain with the start of a run, or the beginning of a basketball or soccer game. The pain tends to work itself out, but by the end of the game or the end of the run, the pain returns. Then the heel may be sore for the rest of the day and the following day.

The treatment is the same as it is listed in Chapter 9. I suggest making some modification to the treatment regimen depending on your pain. Try to incorporate the treatments for the plantar fasciitis and the time spans for treatments for Achilles tendonitis. Both conditions can be difficult to resolve. The longer you have had the problem, the longer it will take for it to go away.

NAIL PROBLEMS

By far, the greatest nail problem encountered by the athlete (most typically the runner) is a *subungual hematoma* (blood under the nail). Although this condition can happen to any one who has an injury to the nail, it commonly happens with repetitive microtrauma. A blood blister develops under the nail, causing a dark brown-black discoloration which becomes painful. This is due to the repetitive pressure at the toes, jamming up against the shoes. This happens more with running down hills, especially those that are steep. The treatment is to place tape directly on the toe-nail (wrapped around the toe) and keep it on throughout the day and throughout exercise. The tape can remain on for days. If you are pulling the tape off and on each day, then place a small piece of gauze on the toenail before taping. This will help to avoid tearing the nail off when you pull the tape off. It is easy for the tape to pull the nail off when you remove it, so be careful. Usually the first one to two weeks, the nail can be loose, but then it will either fall off, or adhere down. If it shows any sign of infection or continues to be painful, have it removed by your doctor. Some doctors will drain the blood from under the nail if it is causing excessive pain or pressure.

Nails will also show unusual changes in shape and color when they are subject to repetitive microtrauma common in running. This may also happen in rock climbing, due to extremely tight shoes. The nails may become brittle, they may become loose or fall off. Sometimes, they become flakey and peel. Here are a few ways to avoid this. First, make sure your shoes fit correctly. You need some room in the toe box for the foot to slide, but too much can lead to problems. If the problem is severe, avoid hills. If you must run hills, run up the steep part and down the part that is not as steep. Taping the nails by wrapping sports tape around the toe and toenail can help when the nails are loose.

BLISTERS

Blisters are a common problem for anyone who is active. They develop as a result of friction that is caused by the shoe rubbing on the sock that rubs on the foot. Any long distance running, walking, jogging, biking, hiking or climbing can result in blisters. Walking in new or rigid shoes can cause blistering. Properly fitting shoes are critical. Properly fitting socks with seams in the appropriate place is another important factor. Don't wear new shoes or rigid shoes on long runs, hikes or walks until they are 'broken in.' If you continue to get blisters, either your shoes are not fitting properly or your socks are not fitting properly. Also, sweating feet can cause an increase in movement of the foot in the shoe and increase friction which can lead to blisters. Increased sweating also leads to cotton socks becoming wet. This can also lead to blister formation. Placing powder in the sock before a run to decrease sweating may help. Also consider thin fleece socks, synthetic socks or thin wool socks. These won't absorb water as much as cotton. Spraying antiperspirant (or using a roll-on) directly on the feet will reduce sweating while running.

If you do have a blister, the best way to treat it is to make a small hole with a sterile needle at the side of the blister. Then drain all the fluid inside. Do not remove the top layer of skin. Place either moleskin or tape directly on the blister and the surrounding area. Make sure the area is dry, and consider using tape adhesive around the edges (not on the blister) to make it stick. Leave the tape and moleskin on for three to five days. Adhesive tape should stay on for that amount of time. Moleskin can become wet in the shower, but if you dry it out before putting on your shoes, it will usually stay on for two to three days. If the tape does come off, peel off carefully; you don't want to remove the roof of the blister. Once the blister is healed, take precautionary measures by placing tape or moleskin at that area before starting the activity again. If you find the tape or moleskin rolling up on the corners, then your skin is either too wet or sweat is not allowing the tape to stick. Tape adhesive will help in these situations. Also consider placing alcohol around the skin area and letting it dry. This will help to dry the skin before application of the tape or moleskin.

> Do not insert needles or pins into your feet if you are diabetic, have poor circulation or you don't have any sensation in your feet.

SHIN SPLINTS

Shin splints are also common in the athlete. The medical term is *tibial periostitis*. They typically develop after increasing the intensity with an activity or starting to walk or run hills. Individuals who play sports involving quick sprints like basketball, soccer or tennis also tend to develop this problem. Typically, the pain is at the front of the shin and the pain occurs with any motion or walking. The pain can also be *palpated* along the shin bone (*tibia*). Rest is typically the best treatment for shin splints. Ice and anti-inflammatory medications

　Those Aching Feet

will also help, but without rest, they will not resolve the problem.

STRESS FRACTURES

Anyone can get a stress fracture, but the athletes are prone to them. A stress fracture is not a full fracture, but a stress in the bone. The long bones in the feet and the tibia (calf bone) are the two that will most commonly give the athlete a problem. Repetitive stress on the foot and leg is the most common cause. Usually, the fracture does not result from an injury, but it can.

A stress fracture in the foot will feel achy and sore. The foot will appear swollen and sometimes bruised. There will be tenderness with any pressure. I recommend low impact or no-impact activity for stress fractures. A rigid soled shoe is necessary for four weeks. The bone will take six weeks to heal, regardless of what treatment you use (and sometimes, for those who do not stay off of their feet, the symptoms can continue for two to three months). Stress fractures do not show up on x-rays for at least two to four weeks after the fracture occurred. I recommend seeking treatment immediately and not pushing your training. There is a chance of developing a full fracture at the point of stress.

ANKLE SPRAINS

Ankle sprains are another common injury for the athlete. Ankle sprains are commonly seen in sports like soccer, basketball, tennis and hiking. The most common ankle sprain occurs on the outside (*lateral*) of the ankle. There are three ligaments that hold the ankle joint in place. When the ankle is twisted, one or more of these ligaments may be torn. Most ankle sprains involve partial tearing of one or more ligaments. Severe ankle sprains involve partial to complete tears of two or three ligaments. The doctor will usually take x-rays to make sure there are no broken bones. There are a few tests the doctor may do, to test for stability.

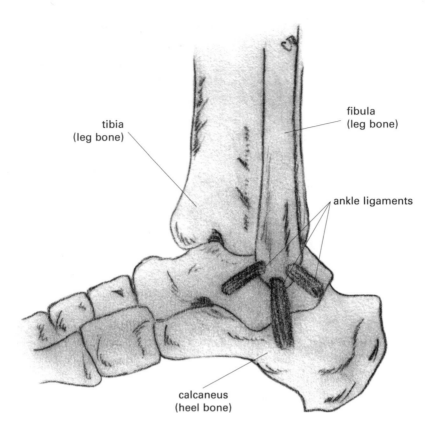

tibia
(leg bone)

fibula
(leg bone)

ankle ligaments

calcaneus
(heel bone)

Figure 14-2 ankle ligaments

A mild to moderate ankle sprain usually involves some moderate swelling and bruising. An aircast or canvas lace-up brace will usually suffice. Very mild ankle sprains may only need an ace bandage and high top shoes. An ankle sprain takes 6-12 weeks to heal, but your return to activity depends on the type of sprain. I recommend seeing your physician. Ice the ankle for three to five days after the injury and stay off of the ankle as much as possible. Use an aircast or lace-up brace for about two weeks. Anti-inflammatory medications (e.g. ibuprofen) may help decrease inflammation during the first week. Do range of motion exercises. Lift your ankle up and down and make circles. A severe ankle sprain requires a cast, usually for four to six weeks, (with crutches to assist walking) and may involve surgery at the time, or after, the initial healing phase. Many times, cast boots are used, so that the boot may be taken off and motion exercises started.

Once you have had a few mild to moderate ankle sprains, or have had one severe ankle sprain, your ankle will be weak. This weakness comes from the ligaments healing in an elongated position. If this results in re-spraining of your ankle five to six times a year, you may need an ankle stabilizing surgery. There are also a few conditions that can result from ankle sprains. One is damage to the cartilage in the ankle joint. This is called a *talar dome* injury. A CT scan is usually needed to diagnose this. It is not common, but if you experience continued ankle pain, long after you have had the injury, this may be a concern. Inflammation of the joint lining of the joint below the ankle joint (at the subtalar joint), is another problem that occurs after ankle sprains. The diagnostic test for this is an injection. Usually the pain feels as if it is at the outside of the ankle and occurs with walking or any activity.

ARTHRITIS

I know what you are thinking, "Why is she including arthritis in the chapter on athletes?" Arthritis can develop with wear and tear, overuse and injury. Athletes put a tremendous amount of stress on their joints and bodies. Any athlete who places excess repetitive stress on their body, has the chance of developing early arthritis. The joints in the body will eventually develop some arthritis, but excess stress or injury may cause change to the joints and eventually arthritis. A common place to develop arthritis in the foot is at the bunion area. If this area is not aligned correctly or one has an extreme flatfoot, early arthritis can develop. After any fracture into a joint, arthritis can develop. This is commonly seen after ankle fractures. Any injury that disrupts the ligaments and damages the cartilage of the joint can lead to early arthritis. There are some treatments for arthritis, but there is no cure for arthritis.

There are some ways to decrease pain. Arthritis occurs when the cartilage in joints starts to wear down. When the cartilage is no longer available as a cushion, bone rubs on bone contributing to the pain of arthritis. The damage to the cartilage is not completely due to wear and tear. Many new theories are relating osteo-arthritis to a breakdown of the cartilage substrate (microscopic layers). In your quest to relieve the pain, try the following treatments:

Contrast soaks
Use alternating hot and cold soaks or you can alternate between hot and cold packs. First place an ice pack on your foot, then switch to a warm pack and finally return to the ice pack. Switch back and forth, using each pack in 5 minutes intervals, for a total of 30 minutes. Ice for 5 minutes, warm for 5 minutes, ice for 5 minutes.

Range of motion exercises
Try this for arthritis and limited motion in your great toe: Soak your toe in warm water for 20 minutes. Then move the toe up and down slowly while pulling the toe out away from the foot. If this increases your pain-stop.

Anti-inflammatories (NSAIDS)
These medications are a good treatment for a short period to decrease the inflammation of an aggravated area. NSAIDS may help decrease the pain at your joint, but they are not the right choice for long term therapy because they are not directed at the problem. There are also potential side effects from prolonged usage.

Appropriate shoes
Certain shoes may be better for those with arthritis. If you have arthritis in your ankle or your great toe joint, then a rigid soled rocker bottom shoe may help decrease the stress through those areas. Comfort is always important, but make sure the shoes are not too flexible. The foot will have to take up this excess stress if the shoe doesn't.

Glucosamine and chondroitin sulfate

These are two supplements that are available at your local drug store. A prescription is not needed. Studies dating back to the 1980's show signs that these two supplements can help relieve the pain of arthritis. These supplements are postulated to enhance the cartilage at a biochemical level. The typical dose of these supplements varies and is usually listed on the label. The recommended dosage is 1,000 mg to 2,000 mg of glucosamine and 800 mg to 1,600 mg of chondroitin sulfate every day. If you can tolerate some medical terminology, I highly recommend reading *The Arthritis Cure* by Jason Theodosakis, M.D., Brenda Adderly, M.H.A. and Barry Fox, Ph.D. This book describes arthritis, its causes, new approaches to treatments and discusses the benefits of glucosamine and chondroitin sulfate.

The Bottom Line

If you participate in sports or are very active, then plan on encountering an injury at one time or another. Act fast when the pain comes on. Stop your usual activity for about five to seven days; cross train instead. Incorporate the therapies listed in this chapter. Rest the foot as much as possible. Ice and stretch twice a day. Slowly ease back into your regular activity over a week. If symptoms persist, see a physician.

SUMMARY

The foot is a very important part of your body and one that is usually neglected. The foot will carry you approximately 75,000-100,000 miles in your life time. The foot absorbs an unbelievable amount of stress and force each day. The average person takes about 8,000 to 10,000 steps a day. A runner may take 2,000 steps in a half hour run. The weight of your body combined with the force of gravity and your leg speed determine the amount of force that goes through your foot with each step. Those 28 bones and 100+ ligaments, combined with the tendons and muscles provide adequate shock absorption and smooth motion.

Taking care of your feet is just as important as taking care of the rest of your body. Usually, eating healthy, exercising regularly and reducing the stress in your life will help not only your body, but your feet as well.

Maintaining a healthy lifestyle is the first step to decreasing pain, aches, weakness and fatigue, especially as you age.

If you can keep your feet from hurting, you'll find that you'll have more energy, and possibly decreased knee and back pain. Remember, the foot is connected to the body. How the foot hits the ground and functions affects the ankles, knees, hips and back. Preventing foot problems by taking care of your feet, identifying foot problems when they arise, and initiating treatments quickly are important steps to having healthy feet. Take care of your feet and they will provide you with many miles of comfortable use.

About the Author

Christine Dobrowolski received her undergraduate degree in biochemistry from the University of California at Davis. She received her Doctorate in Podiatric Medicine (DPM) from The California College of Podiatric Medicine (CCPM). During her residency she trained in foot and ankle surgery. Dr. Dobrowolski has published articles in *The Journal of Foot and Ankle Surgery* and *The Lower Extremity*. She also co-authored a chapter in *The Comprehensive Textbook of Foot Surgery*. She is currently in a private practice in Eureka, California.

Glossary

achilles tendonitis
Inflammation of the achilles tendon that results in pain.

accommodative orthotic
An orthotic that is made to accommodate the foot; made by taking a mold of the foot and using soft material to mold a cushion insert.

acute
Something that develops or happens suddenly.

adductovarus
Rotation of the toe (usually the little toe) inward, towards the big toe.

anesthesia
Can be either local anesthesia or general anesthesia. General

anesthesia involves being put to sleep, having a machine breath for you. Local anesthesia involves having an injection and numbing medication placed into your skin.

anti-inflammatories
Medications taken to decrease inflammation such as ibuprofen.

antibiotic
A medication either taken as a pill, or placed on the skin that will fight infection.

artery
A vessel that carries blood with oxygen and nutrients to the surrounding tissues.

apophysis
The end of a bone in children that allows for growth.

arthroplasty
Surgery that involves removing a joint and straightening the toe.

arthrodesis
Surgery that involves removing the joint, and placing the two bones together so that they don't move. Fusion.

avulsion
Removal of part of the nail or the full nail using a local anesthetic injection to numb the toe. The nail grows back 100% of the time.

benign
Used to describe a mass or tumor when it is not threatening or malignant.

biomechanics
The study of how the muscles, tendons and bones in your body create movement and motion.

biopsied
Taking a small segment of skin or organ and sending it to a pathologist who then examines it under a microscope. At the microscopic level, the pathologist is able to tell if the tissue is benign or malignant.

bunion
Caused by a large bump at the inside of the foot that can result in pain and/or arthritis.

bursa
Sac of fluid that develops in response to pressure to protect a body part or area. There are many anatomical bursas that you are born with and help protect areas of stress.

calcaneal apophysitis
The bony area of the back of the heel that allows for growth in children becomes inflamed. This usually occurs between 8-12 years of age.

calcaneus
The heel bone.

callous
A thickening of skin that usually occurs at areas of pressure or friction. Callouses usually occur on the bottom or at the sides of the feet.

capillaries
The small vessels between the veins and the arteries that allow the oxygen and nutrients to be delivered to the tissues.

capsulitis
Inflammation of the tissue that surrounds the joint.

cardiologist
Heart doctor.

charcot foot
A collapsed foot due to multiple broken bones, usually occurring in a diabetic with no sensation.

circulation
Blood supply to your feet or blood supply traveling away from your feet, to your heart.

conservative treatment
Any treatment done that doesn't involve surgery. The less invasive, the more conservative.

corn
A build up of dead tissue (callous like tissue) usually on the top of the toe or between the toes. Usually a result of a hammertoe.

cuneiforms
Bones in the middle and inside of the foot.

debrided
Removing callous tissue or dead skin with a sharp instrument.

debridements
See debrided.

dermatitis
An inflammation of the skin, usually a reaction to an irritant.

differential diagnosis
Other problems, conditions or diseases that commonly appear like the condition you have.

dorsal bunion
A bump on the top of the big toe joint.

drainage
Fluid that seeps out of a wound or opening in the skin.

endoscopically
Visualizing the inside of the body, with a small camera, through a small incision.

erythrasma
Inflammation between the toes caused by bacteria.

etiology
Cause of a condition or disease.

eversion
See everted.

everted
The position of the foot when it is rolled in with the arch collapsed.

fascia
A structure on the bottom of the foot, similar to a ligament that extends from the heel to the toes.

fibrous
A descriptive medical term for a fiber-like tissue similar to scar tissue.

fixation
Surgical term describing the type of hardware placed in the area to hold two pieces of bone together, such as a screw.

forefoot
The front of the foot which includes the metatarsals (long bones) and the toes.

fracture
Broken bone

functional orthotic
A shoe insert that is made by taking a mold of the foot while it is in a correct position, and then adding corrections to the insert. The insert then holds the foot in a correct position and controls any abnormal motion.

fusion
Joining two bones together in surgery with fixation, so the joint doesn't move.

gait
A style or manner of walking.

ganglionic cyst
A closed sac which develops as an outpouching from a joint or a tendon, usually filled with a jelly like fluid.

general anesthesia
Being put to sleep with injected and inhaled agents, usually during surgery, and having a machine breathe for you.

Haglund's deformity
A bone protuberance at the back of the heel that can be inflamed and cause pain. Usually occurs with high arch feet and with high-heeled shoes. Also called pump-bump.

hammertoe
A crooked toe that cocks up at one joint, and curls under at the next joint.

hammertoe, flexible
A crooked toe that cocks up at one joint, and curls under at the next joint. Will reduce with attempts to manually straighten

hammertoe, rigid
A crooked toe that cocks up at one joint, and curls under at the next joint. Will stay crooked with attempts to straighten.

hyperkeratosis
Dead tissue built up by the body in an area of pressure.

hyperkeratotic tissue
See hyperkeratosis.

hyphae
The spaghetti and meatball appearance of fungus under a microscope.

immunocompromised
The immune system is the part of the body which helps fight

infections. Individuals may be born with or develop a problem with the immune system which subsequently decreases their ability to fight off infection.

immunosuppresive
This usually is referring to an illness or drug's effect on the body. Either of these can "suppress" or decrease the ability of the immune system to function.

incision
Surgical term for cutting the skin during surgery.

inflammation
A combination of redness and swelling to an area.

insertion
A place on the bone where the tendon attaches.

insertional tendonitis
Inflammation of a tendon at it's insertion.

interdigital tinea
Fungus infection of the skin that occurs between the toes.

inversion
See inverted.

inverted
The foot rolling out, with the weight on the outside of the foot and a high arch.

KOH
Potassium hydroxide test that allows for fungus to be observed under the microscope.

lateral
Away from the central line of the body.

ligament
Structure in the body, made mostly of collagen that originates on the bone and inserts on bone and usually crosses a joint.

local anesthesia
Numbing of part of the body with a medication that is injected into the skin.

matrix
The base of the nail, "the root" where the nail grows.

matrixectomy
Permanent removal of all or part of a nail. This is similar to an avulsion except that a chemical is used at the base of the nail, where the nail grows, which causes a chemical burn and prevents the nail from growing back.

medial
Towards the central line of the body.

metatarsal
Long bone in the foot.

metatarsal phalangeal joint, first
The first metatarsal phalangeal joint is the great toe joint. Big toe is a common term for the "great toe".

midfoot
The middle of the foot which contains the cuneiforms, the navicular and the bases of the metatarsals.

MRI
Magnetic resonance imaging. Magnets are used to displace hydrogen atoms in the body, which then emit a signal that is picked up and recorded. The signal varies based on water content. This test is used to see the internal structure of the body.

nail bed
A thickened skin layer under the nail. When the nail grows, it follows the shape of the nail bed.

navicular
A bone in the middle and inside of the foot.

nerve entrapment
A nerve may be caught in scar tissue, rubbed by a tendon or caught in a mass that results in irritation and pain.

neuropathy
Loss of sensation, usually starting with the tips of the toes and moving up the legs. Typically occurs in diabetics.

nodule
A small rounded mass.

onychocryptosis
A nail that is curved in and pinching the skin. It may or may not cause pain and it may or may not cause infection. Commonly referred to as an "ingrown nail".

onychomycosis
A fungal infection of the nails.

orthotics
A custom molded insert that fits into a shoe. Orthotics are made by taking a mold of the foot.

orthotics, functional
Rigid molded inserts designed to control motion.

orthotics, accommodative
Soft molded inserts intended to cushion the foot.

oxidizes
A chemical process involving giving up electrons. An element or radical combining with oxygen.

palpation
Pressing on an area to see if there is pain.

paronychia
An infection that surrounds the nail, usually caused by an ingrown nail.

partial matrixectomy
Permanent removal of only part of the nail. See matrixectomy.

partial nail avulsion
Removing only part of the nail, and allowing it to grow back in. This involves an injection of local anesthetic to numb the toe.

pathologic pes valgus
The medical terminology describing a very severe flatfoot that develops problems as a result.

peroneal tendonitis
Inflammation of the peroneal tendon which runs on the outside of the leg and foot.

pes plano valgus
Medical term for flatfoot.

phalanges
Small bones in the toes.

plantar fascia
A long ligament like structure on the bottom of the foot which starts at the heel and travels out to the toes, holds up about 30% of the arch.

plantar fasciitis
A condition when the long ligament (fascia) on the bottom of the foot develops tears and then becomes inflamed.

posterior tibial tendon
The tendon originates from the muscle which starts in the calf and then as a tendon, courses around the inside of the ankle and attaches at the middle of the arch of the foot.

posterior tibial tendonits
Inflammation of the posterior tibialis tendon, usually where it attaches on the foot. Can be a result of a fallen arch or flatfeet.

pronation
Similar to eversion, but describes a motion, rather than a position. The foot is rolled in, usually with a collapsed arch.

protective threshold

A term used to describe when a person has lost their sensation to a point where an ulceration can form. The body can make adjustments to protect the foot from harm if there is sensation. There is a threshold level, where the amount of sensation that exists is no longer adequate enough to protect the body.

pulses

The arteries in the foot 'pulse' with each heart beat. The two main arteries are on top of the foot and behind the ankle.

rearfoot

The back of the foot, containing the heel bone (calcaneus) the ankle bone (talus) and the cuboid.

retrocalcaneal bursitis

A small sac of fluid at the back of the heel, usually at the attachment of the achilles tendon, can be associated with a heel spur.

retrocalcaneal heel spur

A bone spur at the back of the heel, usually at the attachment of the achilles tendon.

rule out

In order to be sure of a diagnosis, the physician needs to consider the other conditions that appear the same as your condition. Sometimes lab tests are done, or x-rays and other times only more questioning is necessary. Once this is done, the other conditions have been "ruled out".

sebaceous cyst

Soft tissue mass with oily or fatty discharge.

sesamoid

Small bones under the great toe joint, used as lever arms.

stress fracture

Incomplete fracture of the bone.

subungual hematoma
A blood blister that forms under the nail.

supination
Similar to inverted, the foot rolling out with a high arch and more weight on the outside of the foot.

symptom
A feeling your experience as a result of your condition.

synovial cyst
An enclosed sac that forms as an outpouching of a joint, but has a clear, sticky fluid inside (synovial fluid) that lubricates joints.

talar dome injury
Injury to the cartilage and part of the bone under the cartilage in the ankle joint. Can occur as a result of ankle sprains.

talus
Bone in the ankle that sits between the calf bone (tibia) and the heel bone (calcaneus).

tendon
A structure that connects the muscle to the bone.

tibia
Long bone in the calf.

tibial periostitis
The inflammation of the fiber like tissue that lines the bone of the tibia.

tinea pedis
Fungus infection that affects the skin of the feet.

topical
Using a treatment in the form of a cream, a lotion, a liquid a powder on the skin as opposed to taking it by mouth.

ulcer, ulceration
Opening or break in the skin.

vein
Blood vessel that carries blood without oxygen and less body nutrients from the surrounding tissues to the heart.

verrucae
See wart.

vesicular
Small blisters.

vesicular tinea
A fungus infection that presents with peeling, redness and tiny blisters.

vessels
Tubular structures in the body made for carrying blood to and from the heart.

wart
A growth in the skin caused by a virus.

References

Chapter 2: Fungal Nails

Firooz A, et al. **Itraconazole pulse therapy improves the quality of life of patients with toenail onychomycosis.** J Dermatolog Treat 2003 Jun; 14(2): 95-8.

Baran R, et al. **Onychomycosis, the current approach to diagnosis and therapy.** London, Martin Dunitz De Doncker 1999; 6-9.

Gupta AK, et al. **Onychomycosis in children: prevalence and treatment strategies.** J Am Acad Dermtol 1997; 36: 395-402.

Hall M, et al. **Safety of oral terbinafine; Results of a post-marketing surveillance study in 25,884 patients.** Arch Dermatol 1997; 133: 1213-1219.

Pollack R, Billstein S. **Safety of Oral Terbinafine for Toenail Onychomycosis.** JAPMA 1997; (87): 565-570.

De Backer M, et al. **A 12 week treatment for dermatophyte toe onychomycosis: terbinafine 250 mg/day vs. itraconazole 200 mg/day-a double-blind comparative trial**. British Journal of Dermatology 1996; 134(46): 16-17.

Brodell R, et al. **Clinical Pearl: Systemic antifungal drugs and drug interactions**. J Am Acad of Dermatol 1995; 259-260.

Brautigam M, et al. **Randomized double blind comparison of terbinafine and itraconazole for treatment of toenail tinea infection**. British Medical Journal 1995; 311: 919-922.

Idem. **Dermatologic Clinics, The Nails**. Philadelphia, W. B. Sanders Co 1985 Jul; 3(3).

Idem. **Nail changes secondary to systemic drugs or ingestants** JAAD 1984; 10: 250.

Chapter 3: Ingrown Nails

McGlamry ED, Banks SA, Downey SM. *Comprehensive Textbook of Foot Surgery*. Baltimore, William & Wilkins 1992; 289-296.

Yale I. *Podiatric Medicine*. Baltimore, William & Wilkein, 1974; 170-171.

Chapter 4: Foot Fungus

De Doncker P, et al. **Itraconazole pulse therapy for onychomycosis and dermatomycoses: An overview.** J Am Acad of Dermatol 1997; 37(6): 969-973.

Hall M, et al. **Safety of oral terbinafine; Results of a post-marketing surveillance study in 25,884 patients.** Arch Dermatol 1997; 133: 1213-1219.

DeLauro TM, Hodge W. **Dermatophytosis, A review of diagnosis and current therapy.** Clin Pod Med 1986; 3(3): 427-432.

Yale I. *Podiatric Medicine*. Baltimore, William & Wilkin 1974; 132-135.

Chapter 5: Warts

Landsman MJ, et al. **Diagnosis, pathophysiology, and treatment of plantar verrucae.** Clinics in Podiatric Medicine and Surgery 1996; 13(1): 55-71.

Ronna T, Lebwohl M. **Cimetidine therapy for plantar warts.** JAPMA 1995; 85(11): 717-718.

Johnson LW. **Communal showers and the risk of plantar warts.** Journal of Family Practice 1995; 40(2): 136-138.

Landsman MJ, et al. **Carbon Dioxide Laser Treatment of Pedal Verrucae.** Clinics in Podiatric Medicine and Surgery 1992; 9(3): 659-669.

Glover MG. **Plantar warts.** Foot and Ankle 1990; 11(3): 172-178.

McCarthy DJ. **Therapeutic considerations in the treatment of pedal verrucae.** Clin Pod Med 1986; 3(3): 433-448.

Chapter 6: Corns and Callouses

Yale I. *Podiatric Medicine.* Baltimore, William & Wilkin, 1974; 132-135.

Chapter 7: Hammertoes

McGlamry ED, Banks SA, Downey SM. *Comprehensive Textbook of Foot Surgery.* Baltimore, William & Wilkins 1992; 330-336.

Zeringul GN. Harkless, LB. **Evaluation and management of the web corn involving the fourth interdigital space.** JAPMA 1986; 76(4): 210-212.

Gillet, HG **Interdigital clavus: predisposition is the key factor of soft corns.** Clin Orthop 1979 Jul-Aug; (142): 103-9.

Carroll BW, et al. **The two-phalangeal fifth toe. Development, occurrence and relation to heloma durum.** JAPMA 1978; 68(9): 641-645.

Chapter 8: Bunions

McAlindon TE, et al. **Glucosamine and chondroitin for treatment of osteoarthritis** JAMA 2000; 283(11): 1469-1475.

Langman MJ, et al. **Adverse upper gastrointestinal effects of rofecoxib compared with NSAIDS** JAMA 1999; 282(20): 1929-1933.

Peterson WL, Cryer B. **COX-1-Sparing NSAIDS-Is the enthusiasm justified?** JAMA 1999; 282(20): 1961-1963.

Myerson MS. **The etiology and pathogenesis of hallux valgus.** Foot and Ankle Clinics 1997; 2(4): 583-597.

McGlamry ED, Banks SA, Downey SM. *Comprehensive Textbook of Foot Surgery.* Baltimore, William & Wilkins 1992; 469-503.

Dykyj D. **Pathologic anatomy of hallux abducto valgus.** Clinics in Podiatric Medicine and Surgery 1989; 6(1): 1-17.

Cavaliere RG. **New concepts in metatarsal head osteotomies: Reverse buckling techniques.** Clinics in Podiatric Medicine and Surgery 1989; 6(1): 161-178.

Chapter 9: Plantar Fasciitis

Jaivin JS. **The athletic heel.** Foot and Ankle Clinics 1999; 4(4): 865-879.

Singh D, et al. **Plantar Fasciitis.** British Medical Journal. 1997; 315: 172-175.

Pfeffer GB. **Plantar heel pain.** In Baxter DE (ed) *The Foot and Ankle in Sport.* St. Louis, Mosby 1995; 195.

McGlamry ED, Banks SA, Downey SM. *Comprehensive Textbook of Foot Surgery.* Baltimore, William & Wilkins 1992; 431-455.

Schepsis AA, et al. **Plantar fasciitis. Etiology, treatment, surgical results, and review of the literature.** Clinical Orthopedics and Related Research. 1991; 266: 185-196.

Chapter 10: Diabetes

Backonja M, Glanzman RL. **Gabapentin dosing for neuro-pathic pain: evidence from randomized, placebo-controlled clinical trials**. Clin Ther 2003 Jan; 25(1): 81-104.

Horrobin D. **Essential fatty acids in the management of impaired nerve function in diabetes.** Diabetes 1997; 46(2): S90-93.

Ziegler D, et al. **Treatment of symptomatic diabetic periph-eral neuropathy with the anti-oxidant alpha-lipoic acid: A three-week randomized controlled trial (ALADIN Study).** Diabetologia 1995; 38: 1425-33.

Murray HJ, et al. **The pathophysiology of diabetic foot ulcer-ation.** Clin Pod Med 1995; 12(1): 1-15.

Keen H, et al. **Treatment of diabetic neuropathy with gamma linolenic acid.** Diabetes Care 1993; 16: 8-14.

Chapter 11: Flatfeet

Kirb, K. **Biomechanics of the normal and abnormal foot.** JAPMA 2000; 90(1): 30-33.

Munro B, Steele JR. **Household-shoe wearing and purchasing habits. A survey of people aged 65 years and older.** JAPMA 1999; 89(10): 506-514.

Johnson, JE **Pathomechanics of posterior tibial tendon insuf-ficiency** Foot & Ankle Clinics 1997; 2(2): 227-239.

McGlamry ED, Banks SA, Downey SM. *Comprehensive Textbook of Foot Surgery*. Baltimore, William & Wilkins 1992; 769-817.

Chapter 12: Cysts

McGlamry ED. *Comprehensive textbook of foot surgery.* Baltimore, Williams & Wilkins 1992; 1153-1154.

Irving Y. *Podiatric Medicine.* Baltimore, Williams & Wilkins 1974; 207-214.

Chapter 13: Neuroma

McGlamry ED. *Comprehensive textbook of foot surgery.* Baltimore, Williams & Wilkins 1992; 1153-1154.

Irving Y. *Podiatric Medicine.* Baltimore, Williams & Wilkins 1974; 207-214.

Chapter 14: Athletes

McAlindon TE. **Glucosamine and chondroitin for treatment of osteoarthritis.** JAMA 2000; 283(11): 1469-1475.

Perry JR. **Achilles tendon anatomy.** Foot & Ankle Clinics 1997; 2(3): 363-366.

DiGiovanni BF. **Achilles tendonitis and posterior heel disorders.** Foot & Ankle Clinics 1997; 2(3): 411-428.

Clancy WG. **Achilles tendonitis treatment in the athlete.** Foot & Ankle Clinics 1997; 2(3): 429-438.

Forster RF. **Rehabilitation of achilles tendon disorders.** Foot & Ankle Clinics 1997; 2(3): 557-575.

Singh D, et al. **Plantar Fasciitis.** British Medical Journal 1997; 315: 172-175.

Theodosakis J, Adderly B, Fox B. *The Arthritis Cure.* New York, St. Martin's Press 1997; 39-94.

McGlamry ED, Banks SA, Downey SM. *Comprehensive Textbook of Foot Surgery.* Baltimore, William & Wilkins 1992; 431-455.

Schepsis AA, et al. **Plantar fasciitis: Etiology, treatment, surgical results, and review of the literature.** Clinical Orthopedics and Related Research 1991; 266: 185-196.

Index

anti-inflammatory 54, 68, 71, 85, 106, 113-114, 119-122
antibiotics 21
apophysis 111
arch pain 107
arteries 8, 78
arthritis 59, 65, 90, 121-122
arthrodesis 45-46
arthroplasty 45
aspirin 54
athletes 107-109, 115-116, 119, 121
athletic injuries 112

B

baclofen® 85
betadine 23
Bextra® 55
blister 117-118
blood vessels 5, 8, 86
bone spur 21, 39, 74, 99-101, 111
bunion 49-53, 55-56, 58, 90, 103
bunionectomy 57
Burrows® soaks 29
bursa 51, 64, 105, 111

C

calcaneal apophysitis 111
calcaneus 6, 63, 109, 120
callous 33, 37, 39-41, 43, 45, 49, 59, 84, 90
callous tissue 41, 81
calf stretch 116
Canthacur® 35
capsacian 84-85
capsulitis 105
Celebrex® 54-55
charcot foot 91
chondroitin sulfate 123
cimetidine 16, 36
corn 37-41, 43, 45, 84, 90
COX-2 inhibitor 54-55
Crohn's disease 65
cuneiforms 6-7
cyclosporine 16
cyst 100-102

D

Daypro® 54
debridement, debrided 33, 44, 87

hyphae 13
hyphercator 35

I

ibuprofen 53, 68, 120
ice massage 67
immune system 11-12
immunocompromised 11
immunosuppresive 27
inflammation 19, 28, 61-63, 74, 106, 108, 113-115, 121-122
ingrown nail 15, 19-22, 26, 82
injections 21, 24-26
insertional Achilles tendonitis 108
interdigital tinea 28
inversion 9

K

Kerasal®, 41
ketamine 85
ketoprofen 85
KOH 13, 28

L

Lamisil® 15, 28
lateral 8, 49
ligament 5, 7, 46, 61, 104, 120-1, 125
liquid nitrogen 34
Lotrimin® 28
low arch feet 43, 62, 89

M

malignant melanoma 13
matrixectomy 23-24, 26
medial, medially 8, 49, 115
metatarsal 6-7, 39, 46, 49, 51, 54-58, 103-105
microtrauma 14, 19, 116
midfoot 6-7
Mobic® 55
Morton's neuroma 103-105
Motrin® 54

N

nail avulsion 17, 23-24, 26
nail bruising 13
Naprosyn®, 54
navicular 7, 115
nerve 5, 33, 78-80, 103, 105, 111
neuroma 103, 105-106
Neurontin® 85-86

neuropathy 79-81, 83-86, 88
night splints 53, 73
NSAID 54-55, 68, 122

O

onychocryptosis 19
onychomycosis 11
orthopedic surgeon 59
orthotic 41, 52, 70, 72-73, 94, 96-97, 106-107, 114
osteo-arthritis 122

P

palpated 118
palpation 62
paronychia 19
partial nail avulsion 21
pes plano valgus 89, 91
pedorthists 97
Penlac® 15
peroneal tendonitis 115
phalanges 7, 105
phalanx 6-7, 39, 46, 51, 54-57
physical therapy 73
plantar fascia 63, 74
plantar fasciitis 61-62, 65-67, 69, 71, 74, 90, 112-113, 116
podiatrist 24, 40-41, 45, 84, 97
posterior tibial tendonitis 115
posterior tibialis tendonitis 90
prednisone 27
Prexige® 55
pronation 8-9, 40, 49, 52, 62, 91
psoriasis 13-14
psoriatic arthritis 65
pump bump 110

R

Reiter's syndrome 65
Relafen® 54
retrocalcaneal exostosis 65
retrocalcaneal bursitis 111
retrocalcaneal heel spur 111
rheumatoid arthritis 11

S

salicylic acid 34-35
sarcoma 101
sebacious 101
sesamoids 7

shin splints 107, 118
Sporonox® 15
steroid 28, 101
steroid injection 70, 72, 102, 106, 111, 114
stress fracture 119
subtalar joint 121
subungual hematoma 116
supinate, supination 9
surgery 35, 45-47, 55-56, 58-59, 74-75, 96-97, 101-102, 106, 110-111, 115
synovial cyst 101

T

Tagamet® 35-36
talar dome 121
tea tree oil 14
tendon 7, 43, 54-55, 59, 96, 99, 108, 110, 112-115
tendonitis 65, 108-110, 112, 114-115
terfenadine 16
threshold 80
tibia 63, 109, 118, 120
tibial periostitis 118
Tinactin® 28
tinea pedis 27
topical anesthetics 26
Tylenol® 54, 85

U

ulcer 37, 80-82, 87-88, 113
ulceration 47

V

veins 8, 77
verrucae 31
vesicular tinea 28
Vioxx® 54-55

W

wart 31-36, 40

X

x-ray 21, 44, 50, 56-58, 63-65, 88, 100, 104, 119

Z

Zostrix® 84